Social Group Work Today and Tomorrow
Moving from Theory to Advanced Training and Practice

FOURTEENTH ANNUAL SYMPOSIUM ORGANIZING COMMITTEE

ASSOCIATION FOR THE ADVANCEMENT OF SOCIAL WORK WITH GROUPS
Atlanta, Georgia, October 29-November 1, 1992

Chairperson
Benj. L. Stempler

Program Co-Chairs
Marilyn S. Glass
Morris Golden

The Atlanta Planning Group
Bruce Thyer, Abstracts Chair
Dawn Bray and Jane Hamil, Hospitality Co-Chairs
Diane Lewis, Sponsorship Chair
Susan M. Levine, Preregistration Chair
Barbara J. Bower, On-Site Registration Chair
Jane Hamil and Barbara Montgomery, Recognition
and Local Honorees Co-Chairs
Max Casper, Entertainment Chair
Deborah Scopp, Volunteer Coordinator
Barbara Montgomery, Exhibits
Sharlene J. Poticha, Operations Manager
Danielle E. Stempler, Assistant Operations Manager
Judith Palais, Special Services

Committee Participants

Narviar C. Barker
Harvey Bertcher
Nance Bogardts
Gale Bogart
Janet Cronwell
Paul H. Ephross
Howard Epstein
James A. Garland

Rosalyn Hosenball
Nancy Loeb
John H. Ramey
Jim Sacco
Kathryn Smith
John Templeton
Naomi Ward

Social Group Work Today and Tomorrow
Moving from Theory to Advanced Training and Practice

Benj. L. Stempler, MSW, BCD
Marilyn S. Glass, MA, LPC
Editors

With Christine M. Savinelli, MSW

The Haworth Press
New York • London

Selected Proceedings of the Fourteenth Symposium on Social Work with Groups, Atlanta, Georgia.

The Haworth Press, Inc., 10 Alice Street, Binghamton, NY 13904-1580

Library of Congress Cataloging-in-Publication Data

Social group work today and tomorrow : moving from theory to advanced training and practice / Benj. L. Stempler, Marilyn S. Glass, editors.
    p.   cm.
  Includes bibliographical references and index.
  ISBN 0-7890-6023-X (alk. paper)
  1. Social group work. I. Stempler, Benj. L. II. Glass, Marilyn S.
HV45.S617 1996
361.4–dc20
                                                    96-359
                                                    CIP

This book is dedicated to Dr. Robert Salmon and the late Dr. Florence S. Schwartz, whose patient guidance and gifted teaching gave me the road map to start me on my way, and to my wife and daughter, Sharlene and Dani, whose love and support have enabled me to complete this phase of the journey.

Benj. L. Stempler

CONTENTS

Foreword   xvii
        James A. Garland

Preface   xxi
        Benj. L. Stempler

Acknowledgments   xxv

**Chapter 1. Social Work with Groups: Paradigm Shifts
for the 1990s**   1
        Lawrence Shulman

Introduction   1
Paradigms and Paradigm Shifts   1
The Medical Paradigm   2
An Oppression Model and Social Work Practice   5
The Interactional Paradigm   7
Conclusion: Group Work's Contribution to the Shift
   in the Social Work Paradigm   16

**Chapter 2. Making Joyful Noise: Presenting,
Promoting, and Portraying Group Work
to and for the Profession**   19
        Roselle Kurland
        Robert Salmon

**Chapter 3. AIDS and Group Work: Looking
into the Second Decade of the Pandemic**   33
        George S. Getzel

Objectives   34
Personal Perspective   34
An Uncertain Condition   35
Crisis Situation   36
Identity Concerns   37

Theoretical Perspective 38
Rites of Passage 38
Rationale for Groups 39
Life Cycle Re-Enactment 41
Legacy and Identity 42
The Future 42

Chapter 4. Positive Group Work Experiences with African-American Adolescents 1935-1945: An Afrocentric Retrospective Analysis 45

Marjorie Witt Johnson

Self-Concept/Skin Color 47
Early Dance Group Experiences 48
Processes: Decision Making and Personal Interaction 49
Termination of the Group 53
Recommendations 54

Chapter 5: The New Patient Mix: Group Work and Chronic Disorders in an Acute Care Hospital 57

Patricia Moffat
Noreen Kay

The Setting 57
The New Patient Mix 57
Relative Growth of Three Groups of Elderly 58
Who is Helping Community Residents 55 and Older? 59
Social and Lifestyle Factors in Elder Care 60
Social Group Work in Health Care 60
Three Groups Work Approaches in Acute Care 61
A Health Education Group for Diabetics 62
Cardiac Spouses: A Support Group with Staff Education
    Features 64
Enhancing Competency and Mutual Support: A Staff Group
    in Oncology 67
Conclusions 68

Chapter 6. Bringing the Mountain to Mohammed: An Experiential Approach to Teaching Group Dynamics in the Classroom　　71

Marcia B. Cohen

Educational Setting and Course Assignment　　72
Roles　　73
Norms　　76
Interactional Patterns　　79
Group Development　　81
Student Evaluations of the Task Group Experience　　83
Conclusion　　84

Chapter 7. Social Group Work with Recovering Women: An Empowerment Model　　87

Rita Rhodes
Ann Johnson

Morality Model　　87
Medical Model　　88
Ecological Model　　91
An Empowerment Model of Group Work　　93
Crisis Work　　94
Value of Group Experience for Women　　94
Content　　95
Implications for Social Work Practice　　99

Chapter 8. Redefining Adult Identity: A Coming Out Group for Lesbians　　103

Anna Travers

Lesbians, Homophobia, and the Coming Out Process　　103
Identity Issues for Lesbians Who Are Coming Out　　105
The Appropriateness of Group Work　　107
Composition of the Group　　110
Group Structure and Content　　111
Group Process Issues　　114

Chapter 9. Being Non-Deliberative on "A Hot Winter's Night": Confessions of a Creative Practitioner   **119**

Paul Earl Rivers

Substantive Issue   119
Social Work Practice Episode   120
Major Features of this Form of Practice   121
Non-Deliberative Theoretical Connections   122
Conclusion   125

Chapter 10. Trauma Debriefings: A One-Session Group Model   **129**

Tom Reynolds
Gwyn Jones

Stages of a Trauma Debriefing Model   131
  Pre-Group Activity   131
  Beginning Phase   132
  The Middle Phase   134
  The Ending Phase   136
  Post-Group Phase   137
Conclusion   137

Index   **141**

ABOUT THE EDITORS

Benj. L. Sempler, MSW, BCD, is Managing Associate at the Atlanta Center for Group Work & Psychotherapy and is an independent clinical social worker in Atlanta, Georgia. Prior to holding these positions, he was Clinical Social Worker for the Jewish Family Services, Inc., for ten years. The Chairperson of the Fourteenth Annual Symposium on Social Work with Groups in 1992, he is the author of several articles and papers on group work approaches to social work. He was Chairperson of the Georgia Chapter Development Committee of the Association for the Advancement of Social Work with Groups from 1988 until 1992 and the President of that organization from 1992 to 1994. Mr. Stempler is a member of the American Association for Marriage and Family Therapists and the Academy of Certified Social Workers.

Marilyn S. Glass, MA, LPC, is an independent practitioner in Atlanta, Georgia. With more than 25 years of experience as a therapist and teacher, she works with individuals, couples, and groups. Her particular interest in women, their development and their relationships, has led to her recent work with women's support groups. This work has reaffirmed her belief in the power of group work for increasing understanding and supporting change. A member of AASWG, Ms. Glass served as Chair of the Continuing Education Committee for the Georgia Chapter from 1992 to 1994.

Editorial Associate

Christine Savinelli, MSW, is a graduate of the Boston University School of Social Work. After obtaining an MSW, Ms. Savinelli relocated to Atlanta, Georgia and became involved with the Georgia chapter of AASWG. At that time, her interest and dedication to social work with groups continued to grow. She was employed at a private psychiatric hospital in which she was primarily involved in group work with children and adolescents. Ms. Savinelli moved back to her home state of Connecticut in January, 1995. She is currently employed as a Psychiatric Social Worker at the Adolescent and Children's Crisis Unit for Treatment and Evaluation (ACCUTE), in New Haven, CT. She provides out-patient crisis assessment intervention services as well as in-patient psychiatric care at a nearby hospital. Ms. Savinelli is anxious to become involved in social work with groups in the near future.

CONTRIBUTORS

Marcia B. Cohen, PhD, University of New England School of Social Work, Biddeford, ME.

George S. Getzel, DSW, Professor, Hunter College School of Social Work, New York, NY.

Ann Johnson, MSW, Richland Memorial Hospital, Columbia, SC.

Marjorie Witt Johnson, MSW, ACSW, Consultant, Group Work and the Arts, Cleveland Public Schools, Cleveland, OH.

Gwyn Jones, MSW, Regional Clinical Director, Warren Sheppell Consultants Corp., Toronto, Canada.

Noreen Kay, MSW, CSW, Social Work Team Leader, Surgery Team, Sunnybrook Health Science Centre, University of Toronto, Toronto, Canada.

Roselle Kurland, PhD, Hunter College School of Social Work, New York, NY.

Patricia Moffat, MSW, CSW, Social Work Supervisor, Baycrest Centre for Geriatric Care, Toronto, Canada; Group Work Consultant, Sunnybrook Health Science Centre, University of Toronto, Toronto, Canada.

Tom Reynolds, MSW, CSW, Senior Manager, EAP Services, The Bank of Montreal, Toronto, Canada.

Rita Rhodes, PhD, Assistant Professor, University of South Carolina, College of Social Work, Columbia, SC.

Paul Earl Rivers, MSW, Toronto Hospital, Western Division Department of Social Work, Toronto, Canada.

Robert Salmon, Professor, DSW, Hunter College School of Social Work, New York, NY.

Lawrence Shulman, Professor, Boston University School of Social Work, Boston, MA.

Anna Travers, MSW, Shout Clinic, Toronto, Canada.

Symposia Chairpersons:

John H. Ramey, 1991 (see General Secretary above).

Benj. L. Stempler, 1992, Atlanta Center for Group Work and Psychotherapy, Atlanta, GA.

Robert Salmon, 1993, School of Social Work, Hunter College, New York, NY.

Roselle Kurland, 1993, School of Social Work, Hunter College, New York, NY.

At-Large Members:

Toby Berman-Rossi
Margot Breton
Max Casper
Anita E. Curry-Jackson
Maeda J. Galinsky
Alex Gitterman

Lorraine Guitierrez
Lillian C. Kimura
Nazneen S. Mayadas
Sally Ann Shields
Celia B. Weisman
Bernard J. Wohl

Chapter Representatives:

Margot Breton, Toronto
Catherine G. Corton, CT
Bonnie J. Engelhardt, MA
Hans S. Falck, VA
Morris Golden, GA
Patricia Gulino, FL

Gerald A. Halper, NJ
Lisa E. McGuire, IN
Florence Mittwoch, Israel
Joan K. Parry, No. CA
Thomas G. Ruhala, Mid-MI

Joint Commission on Standards and Linkages for Group Work Practice and Education:

Joan K. Parry
Lawrence Shulman

Representative Emerita:

Beulah G. Rothman (deceased)

Life Members:

Catherine A. Papell
Martin L. Birnbaum

Foreword

This collection of lively and well-written articles was selected from among the presentations made at the Fourteenth Annual Symposium on Social Work with Groups in Atlanta, Georgia in 1992. Focusing on content that speaks to present-day practice and conceptual issues, editors Benj. L. Stempler and Marilyn S. Glass have achieved diversity in authorship, setting, geographical region (albeit comprising only the USA and Canada), and client background.

Group types and formats range from verbal to activity; from one session to beyond one year; from education to support; and from developmental to rehabilitation. Ethical, self-esteem, identity, and empowerment themes are prominent throughout the collection and are in keeping with the historic emphases of social group work as they are reflected in the 1990s context. Client ages identified range from adolescent to aging. Only children, per se, are not represented; a condition regrettably familiar in the group work literature and professional education in general.

The lead articles, both plenary presentations at the Symposium, strike a strong note for social group work's base in an interactionist perspective and for the overall efficacy and uniqueness of the method. Lawrence Shulman's discussion of paradigm shifts from medical to mutual aid endorses derigidification of the worker's stance and spontaneity as an alternative to formality and objective neutrality. His use of a record of service with a group of adults diagnosed with schizophrenia illustrates how a competency and empowerment approach enables them to achieve dignity and normal functioning, although the analysis may have thrown out the psychodynamic baby with the medical bath. Roselle Kurland and Robert Salmon urge us to "make a joyful noise" about social group work and take pride in our historical technology and values. They emphasize that fun, playfulness, and action methods should be "owned" by us and spoken, taught, and written about as we engage in the advocacy, educational reform, and education of our students. Taken together, the two presentations make an affirming and inspirational introduction for what follows.

George S. Getzel continues his already moving and wise series of studies on group work and HIV/AIDS, with an analysis of the second decade of the pandemic. His distressing account of the "mass slaughter" and its effect on its victims, their loved ones, and their caregivers is followed by his characteristically personal recounting of the "special demands on persons who face the consequences of AIDS in their daily living. . . . " He presents a summary of group work approaches and risks, general theoretical implications for AIDS and other kinds of group work, and a perspective for the future.

Marjorie Witt Johnson, a pioneer in developmental and culture-based group work, recounts her decades-long work with African-American adolescents, using her learning of her own heritage and her background in dance to imbue self-worth, confidence, and pride in her young group members. She turned in recent years to formal study of social group work theory to discover whether she was "on the right track" (personal communication). How admirable she was and is, is illustrated in her article. Readers of this volume are encouraged to consult the group work archives to experience her method and personal style as revealed on a video that was made of her presentation.

Patricia Moffat's account of group work with a "new patient mix" in an acute care hospital, offers an impressive description and analysis of how chronic disorders among elderly clients in this decade present an array of life dilemmas and challenges for care. How well a hospital system can reorganize to institutionalize differential group services for this diverse population is seen in Moffat's review and makes this ground-breaking effort must reading for similarly employed professionals.

The dilemmas of caregiving institutions that have not made such progress with group work and that are constantly not able to offer "live" group experiences to social work students, served as the stimulus that impelled Marcia B. Cohen and her colleagues to "bring the mountain to Mohammed" by creating a system for providing simulated practice group experiences as part of the graduate curriculum. This chapter indicates the values and limits of employing a model featuring self-directed student groups and practitioner/instructor consultants.

Rita Rhodes and Ann Johnson present an empowerment model for helping women in recovery that transcends older, moral, and medically based Alcoholics Anonymous (AA) approaches. Based on an ecological analysis of the multiple variables associated with continuing substance abuse this ongoing sobriety intervention, like most of the work presented in this book, relies on mutual aid, self-esteem-producing problem solving, and "feelings work."

In a similar affirmative vein, Anna Travers, in her work with lesbians who are coming out, moves beyond traditional explanations and approaches to focus on the redefinition of adult identity. Emphasizing that these are not psychotherapy groups, Travers helps women discover and redefine themselves through the use of the small group as a microsociety.

Returning to the HIV/AIDS arena, this time in an educational mode, Paul Earl Rivers describes groups for adult gay men that include both learning about, as well as "eroticizing" safer sex practices. Various non-deliberative forms (e.g., games, role play, creative writing), as well as direct information giving, are emphasized. Rivers does not deal with some process issues, such as the pace of being acquainted, extra-group member contacts, context of service program, if any, and other supports, if required.

Tom Reynolds and Gwyn Jones present a dramatic and innovative ending to the volume in their description of a one-session group in a workplace setting to debrief employee-clients concerning traumatic experiences on the job. The context and format include: (1) proprietary service providers; (2) a variety of commercial, non-clinical, and private employer settings; (3) time-limited, circumscribed interventions; (4) use of manuals, non-traditional terminology (e.g., debriefing); and (5) close involvement of business managers in the process. This is the closest any of these offerings has come to the "managed care world." Correspondingly, the reader will note that several issues, such as confidentiality, members' traumatic histories, pre- and post-meeting interviews, manager's role, and positive versus negative pre-group member connections, are, if at all, minimally addressed. This item, like the other material contained between these covers, offers food for thought.

Taken together, Georgia 1992 offered a feast of problems and solutions, reaffirmations and challenges, and new methods and new questions. The Association for the Advancement of Social Work with Groups (AASWG) is grateful to the Georgia colleagues for that experience, and to Benj. L. Stempler and Marilyn S. Glass, and to the authors for this representative selection and its excellent portrayal of the continuing evolution of social group work.

James A. Garland, LICSW
President, AASWG (1991-1994)
Boston University
School of Social Work

Preface

The Fourteenth Annual Symposium on Social Work with Groups was born out of a casually dropped suggestion at an AASWG Chapter Development Committee meeting in Montreal in October 1989. Little did I know when I suggested Atlanta would be a good place to hold a symposium, that it would be acted upon so quickly by AASWG's board. Yet two days later, upon returning from dinner, I was advised that Atlanta had been awarded the symposium, either in 1991 or 1992, and that I was to be the future symposium chairperson. Thus began a task that culminated three years later at Atlanta's Marriott Marquis Hotel and may one day be completed.

In being asked to act also as the senior editor of this volume of proceedings, I found myself confronted with a dual directional task that felt almost as monumental as directing the staging of the Fourteenth Symposium. First, I needed to choose only ten papers from the more than 50 manuscripts submitted (out of almost 80 presented papers) for consideration. Second, I had to examine the papers both from their literary value to the field of social group work, while also attempting to have these selections reflect the overall theme of *Social Group Work Today and Tomorrow: Moving from Theory to Advanced Training and Practice.* It is our hope and belief that the following ten articles reflect the quality and theme of the Atlanta Symposium.

In paring down the many excellent submissions we received, the intent of my co-editor, Marilyn S. Glass, LPC, and I was to reflect the contributions of not only the "giants" of social group work, but also to recognize the contributions of the current generation of educators and practitioners. We also wanted to reflect the Symposium's subtopic areas of theory, education and training, practice, and research. Although in the end there were no pure research papers, we do believe that the quality of the efforts throughout the papers reflects the research of others in their final versions.

We have opened the book with three papers, the first of which was based upon Lawrence Shulman's Keynote address on paradigms for the 1990s, an interactionist theoretical perspective as a means for looking toward creative uses of group work for the future. This is followed by Roselle Kurland's and Robert Salmon's plenary address, the theme of which was to encourage all of us involved with groups–educators, students, and practitioners, to "make a joyful noise." Then comes George Getzel's touching, sad, and moving chapter, based upon his invitation presentation on the second decade of the (AIDS) pandemic.

We then turned to Marjorie Witt Johnson, a group work elder, but "young" author, who wrote of her creative use of dance and group work together, more than 40 years before, based on her work with African-American adolescents. Moving from working with the young to responding to the needs of the ill elderly, Patricia Moffat and Noreen Kay present another example of the use of creative group work with a challenging population. This chapter is followed by Marcia B. Cohen's writing of her efforts in developing creative "practice groups" for her students to help prepare them to work with groups upon their graduation to the ranks of social work professionals.

The next two chapters both address women's issues and empowerment. The first by Rita Rhodes and Ann Johnson, an educator and practitioner, respectively, shows how group work can effectively support women in recovery from substance abuse. The second chapter by Anna Travers is based upon her work to support lesbian women in "coming out," in a way that is affirming. Anna is new to the symposium stage and her very meaningful work is reflective of the effort to identify and validate the latest generation of group workers.

Paul Earl Rivers, another of this newest group-work generation, offers the second HIV-themed chapter in the collection. In his writings, he addresses creative ways to use groups to educate safe sexual practices among homosexual men. Finally, to close the volume is the work of Tom Reynolds and Gwyn Jones. They explore the use of one-session groups or collectivities in the workplace as an effective means for responding to job-related trauma. In choosing this paper, we were responding to the rapidly growing need to apply group work theory to practice in an increasingly time-limited and managed-care oriented society.

In closing, we believe this book is an accurate reflection of the quality, creativity, and energy that made up the Fourteenth Symposium. We are appreciative of the efforts of the authors contained herein and all the presenters who contributed to the unique nature of AASWG's 1992 showcase of the best social group work has to offer. We feel confident that the creativity and innovativeness present at the Atlanta Symposium and reflected by these selected proceedings will offer ideas and direction to all of you who choose to experience the joy of working with groups.

Benj. L. Stempler, MSW, BCD
Chairperson
Fourteenth Annual Symposium
on Social Work with Groups

Acknowledgments

The editors would like to acknowledge all of the presenters and participants at the Fourteenth Symposium; the support and patience of the authors who contributed to this volume; the educational co-sponsors (Clark-Atlanta University School of Social Work, Georgia State University Department of Social Work, and the University of Georgia School of Social Work); the past chairpersons of AASWG Symposias; the past editors of AASWG Symposia Proceedings; and the entire membership of AASWG and GAASWG, their officers and board members, without whom there would not have been a Fourteenth Symposium in Atlanta, Georgia, or a reason for this volume to have been written.

We also would like to acknowledge the superb staff of Atlanta's Marriott Marquis Hotel, especially Rebecca Patterson, Bruce Winter, Bob Walsh, and Larry Fazioli, who made the impossible happen from October 28 to November 1, 1992.

We would also like to acknowledge all of the many volunteers of the Fourteenth Symposium, with a special mention to the BSW students from Concord College, Athens, West Virginia, who came through above and beyond anything we could have imagined.

Finally, we acknowledge James A. Garland, Paul H. Ephross, Patricia Gulino, John H. Ramey, and Carol Ramey, whose wisdom and guidance were invaluable from October 1989 through to the present and, we hope, beyond it.

Thank you all.

Chapter 1

Social Work with Groups: Paradigm Shifts for the 1990s

Lawrence Shulman

INTRODUCTION

As the social work profession enters the last decade of the century it is undergoing fundamental changes. The paradigms that guide professional practice are shifting. Social work with groups, one of the three foundation methods that make up the trinity of practice (casework, group work, and community organization), has played an important role in transforming the way we think about clients and about the helping process. This chapter discusses these paradigm shifts and some of the resultant changes. In addition, the discussion suggests some unique elements associated with social work practice with groups, which may explain why it has played a unique role in this rethinking of the way we work. First, the term *paradigm* and the concept of a *paradigm shift* is explained and illustrated.

PARADIGMS AND PARADIGM SHIFTS

The term *paradigm* is used in this discussion as it was described by Kuhn (1962) in his book on the process of change in scientific

This chapter is based upon the keynote presentation at the Fourteenth Annual Symposium of the Association for the Advancement of Social Work with Groups, October 1992, Atlanta, Georgia.

theory development. He described a paradigm as including the models, theories, and research approaches that guide a discipline in its pursuit of knowledge. Within a single paradigm there could be many different theories; however, all would be guided by the basic framework to which most, if not all, scientists in the discipline subscribe. In one illustration, he described the paradigm that dominated astronomy in its early stages. This paradigm, developed by Ptolemy, suggested that the earth was the center of the universe. Kuhn described how Galileo and Copernicus shifted the guiding paradigm by advocating a new model that placed our sun at the center of the universe. In turn, the Copernican paradigm was replaced by later shifts that enhanced the ability of astronomers to explain the universe (e.g., Newton, Einstein, and the more recent models). Social work, as well as other helping professions, is experiencing its own fundamental paradigm shifts.

THE MEDICAL PARADIGM

Social work adopted a paradigm early in its development. This model was borrowed from the medical profession, considered to be a high-status, successful profession (Shulman, 1991, 1992). The medical paradigm described practice as a three-stage, linear process. First, the professional would conduct a study designed to obtain information about the client's current life, and often about the client's family history as well. In the second stage, the professional, often with the help of a supervisor or team, would use the information to develop a diagnosis or assessment. The client might be involved in this stage, contributing to the identification of the problem. In the third stage, the diagnosis would form the basis of an initial treatment plan to be implemented with the cooperation of the client. Evaluation of treatment outcomes was added as a fourth stage designed to feed information back into the study process, which might lead to a revision in the diagnosis and alternative treatment strategies. This medical paradigm helped social work to move from the "friendly visitor" (Richmond, 1918) phase of its development to a more professional model. Each of the elements of the paradigm–study, diagnosis, treatment, and evaluation–will always be central to our work.

It is not the separate elements themselves but rather the linear nature of the three-stage model that requires reconsideration. When the social work profession adopted this paradigm, it also accepted a number of associated assumptions that have increasingly come into question as our practice and research have altered our understanding of the nature of helping. For example, a social worker engaged in the study phase during a first group session is already well into the treatment process. The group leader's questions, empathy, display of interest, and concern in the members, and the group members' recognition that they are "all in the same boat" have started the healing process. A linear, three-stage paradigm that describes treatment as following study and diagnosis does not adequately describe this more dynamic process. The use of this paradigm as a model can easily lead a novice group worker to focus on "information gathering" in first sessions while ignoring the important, therapeutic processes initiated in the engagement phase.

Another potential problem associated with the medical paradigm is the suggestion that the group leader is the "expert" who can provide a "solution" once the problem is properly diagnosed. This model may minimize the importance of mutual aid and the recognition that the most important help comes not from the leader, but from the members themselves. An alternative paradigm would suggest that the group leader is not an expert in life but rather an expert in helping group members to create, develop, and maintain mutual aid systems. This idea is often commonly described as an "empowerment" model that had its roots in group work practice.

The medical paradigm may also lead the professional to take responsibility for determining what problem or issue should be dealt with in each session. Thus, the group leader feels that he or she "owns" the group and it should be used for the professional's therapeutic purposes. One consequence of this approach is that the group leader takes over the work of the group by developing "goals" for each session, sometimes in consultation with a supervisor or team. In reality, the group members' sense of urgency should determine the focus of the session, and a group leader intent on achieving his or her own goals may completely miss the indirect cues at the start of a session signalling the clients' agenda.

In one classic videotape, which was part of my early research

(Shulman, 1981), a young woman was talking with a social worker in a room with only a video camera present. The client had given permission for the videotaping as part of the research project, but did not know the researcher (this author) who would view the tape. The young woman made repeated attempts to raise through indirect means a problem related to sex. Each effort was missed by the worker, who though attentive, was busy pursuing her own written agenda for the session. The hints became stronger. Fifteen minutes into the session, the client turned to the camera, and in an exasperated tone, asked: "Do you understand?" In this research, when 120 hours of individual and group sessions were videotaped and analyzed using a category observation system developed by this author, this lack of "sessional contracting" was observed as group leaders appeared to be working on one agenda while the clients were sending signals of another–each missing each other.

Finally, another potential problem associated with the use of the medical paradigm is the tendency to rely on a pathology or illness orientation for making assessments. In this diagnostic framework, an emphasis is placed on what is wrong with the client and what needs to be changed. For example, teenage mothers might be judged as inadequate and referred to a parenting group in order to "teach them effective parenting skills." The focus of the group discussion might be on helping the parents better understand their children's needs for "quality time" and parental support. An agenda for discussion and presentations might be designed to teach a curriculum for effective parenting. Many of the group members may be attending because their child-welfare-protection social worker suggested it could be helpful for them if they wished to keep or regain custody of their child. Group sessions of this type often create an illusion of work with clients learning to say what they think their group leader wants to hear as opposed to what they really think and feel.

The medical model as a diagnostic approach has been challenged by many new and emerging frameworks (e.g., strength model, ecological framework, feminist psychology). More recently, a unifying theme focusing on oppression and vulnerability has been articulated. One version of the oppression model will be illustrated in the next part of this chapter.

This same group of teen mothers when viewed from a "strength" perspective might be seen as showing incredible determination and backbone for wanting to keep their children. A support group with this orientation would start with the assumption that these mothers need help from the workers and each other in reinforcing their determination and developing strategies for coping. The same mothers viewed from an ecological model (Germain and Gitterman, 1980) would be best understood as experiencing a conflict between the normative developmental needs of their children and their own needs as teenagers. Discussion might focus on what formal and informal support systems can help them to deal with the absence of a "goodness of fit" between their needs and those of their children.

At this point, it is important to note the difference between the terms *medical model* and *medical paradigm*. The term *medical model,* as just described, refers to an assessment framework that may make up one element of the medical paradigm. The term *medical paradigm,* as used here, refers to the overarching, three-step model of the helping process (study, diagnosis, and treatment). It is entirely possible for a group leader to abandon the medical model as a diagnostic orientation and yet still practice within the medical paradigm. For example, a social worker may use a strength orientation for understanding the group members while still conceiving of the helping process as one in which diagnosis follows assessment and is then followed by treatment.

In the next section, an oppression model for assessment is presented as an alternative to the medical model. This model provides a framework that fits more comfortably into the interactional paradigm—described in more detail in a later section.

AN OPPRESSION MODEL
AND SOCIAL WORK PRACTICE

Frantz Fanon, an early exponent of the psychology of oppression, was a black, West Indian revolutionary psychiatrist (Buhlan, 1985). Whereas Fanon's work emerged from his observations of white-black oppression associated with the efforts of European colonial powers to economically exploit third-world countries, many of his insights and constructs can be generalized to other forms of oppression. While the complete exposition of his views is more complex than presented here, the central idea of gaining one's sense of self through the exploitation of others can be seen in different oppressive relationships and takes many forms: (1) the abusing parent and the abused child; (2) the battering spouse and his partner; (3) male-female sexism; (4) the scapegoating of religious, ethnic, and racial groups; (5) the "abled" population and the "differently abled"; (6) the "normal" population and the "mentally ill"; and (7) and the straight society's oppression of gay men and lesbian women. In all of these examples, one group (usually the majority) uses another group for enhancing a sense of self.

Repeated exposure to oppression, subtle or direct, may lead vulnerable members of the oppressed group to internalize the negative self–images projected by the external oppressor–the "oppressor without." The external oppressor may be an individual (e.g., the sexual abuser of a child) or our society (e.g., the racial stereotypes perpetuated about people of color). Internalization of this image and repression of the rage associated with oppression may lead to destructive behaviors toward self and others as oppressed people become "autopressors," participating in their own oppression. Thus, the oppressor from without becomes the oppressor within. Evidence of this process can be found in the maladaptive use of addictive substances and the growing internal violence within communities of oppressed people, such as we are witnessing in our inner cities.

If we consider the group of teenage mothers described in the previous section, then an oppression framework might focus on the various forms of oppression that these young women have experienced. All of them have experienced some form of gender or racial oppression. As children, some may have experienced physical, emotional or sexual abuse. The internalized negative self-image (the "oppressor within") is fostered as these same women experience the economic oppression associated with poverty. With this perspective in place, one quickly can identify the strengths that have been required to help these young women simply survive. A parents group may help them develop the skills associated with effective parenting, but the orientation of the oppression model would be toward helping them identify and freeing themselves from the internalizations that have blocked their ability to be supportive of their children. The focus of the work is not on the pathology of the women, but rather on helping them develop more adaptive ways of coping with the psychological and emotional impact of long-term and persistent oppression. The group would attempt to deal with the needs of the parents, which, in turn, will provide help for the children.

Buhlan (1985), who chronicled Fanon's life and focused on his psychology, identified several key indicators for objectively assessing the degree of oppression. Whereas Fanon's work explored these indicators in the context of slavery, Buhlan suggests that "All situations of oppression violate one's space, time, energy, mobility, bonding, and identity" (p. 124). Consider these six indicators (Buhan credits the first four items of this list to Chester M. Pierce) as you read the process recording excerpts in the next section taken from a discussion by mentally ill patients on a psychiatric ward.

THE INTERACTIONAL PARADIGM

The argument advanced in this chapter is that the helping professions are experiencing a fundamental shift in the paradigms that guide our practice. The shift to an oppression perspective for assessing clients is just one element of this broader change. This change illustrates Kuhn's (1962) suggestion that an alternative paradigm must be available before a discipline will give up the old one. The *interactional paradigm* offers one alternative method for organizing our thinking about the helping process. It incorporates the elements that have always been important to our practice, but organizes them in a manner that departs from the linear, three-stage model. In addition, it fits well with the oppression model described in the previous section.

A number of core elements from the interactional paradigm are described and illustrated in this section: (1) *understanding the dynamic interaction between the group and the environment;* (2) *responding to the productions of the group members;* (3) *integrating one's personal and professional selves;* (4) *understanding the group as a dynamic system;* and (5) *the social worker's responsibility for the two clients.*

The process recording excerpts used as illustrations are drawn from the work of a social work student with a group of 40- to 65-year-old, white, male veterans, primarily working class from various ethnic groups. All of the men have a diagnosis of chronic schizophrenia and are institutionalized on a psychiatric ward. Many of the concepts of the oppression model, introduced earlier, can readily be applied to the institutionalized mentally ill population. In the excerpts that follow, it is not difficult to perceive violations of institutionalized patients' space, time, energy, mobility, bonding, and identity.

The student noted the heavy load of mandated "therapy" and "living" groups on the ward and decided to offer a voluntary, task-focused group with the purpose of developing and publishing a patient newsletter. These mandated groups could be viewed as two indicators of oppression–violations of time and energy. The student's assessment of the problem demonstrated her understanding of the interactional paradigm *principle of the dynamic interaction between the group and the environment*–in this case, the hospital system. She also communicated her clear sense of her social work role.

The task this group faces is one of negotiating the larger system in which it is situated in order to produce a patient newsletter. Some of the challenges faced by the group are the resistance from the larger system (the hospital), resistance within the group (fear of making waves), members' fear of retribution from staff, feelings of disempowerment, and suspicion from inside and outside of the group. The major problem then, as I see it, is the feeling of disempowerment embodied by the group members. This is illustrated by the reluctance to express themselves honestly in the newsletter. A second, related problem is the hospital's low expectations of the patients and the ambivalence of the hospital toward change. The problem I face is to find a way of mediating between these two systems.

Several incidents occurred which led to this assessment. When I began the newsletter, I observed a great deal of enthusiasm initially, both from group members and staff, but this enthusiasm began to falter after the first few meetings. Many of the members failed to complete the assignments they had volunteered for, and the promised support from the outside system was not forthcoming. Staff members discussed the need to censor the newsletter before it was distributed, a process that heightened and reinforced group member's fears and reservations. I realized that some of these issues would need to be addressed if the group were to proceed any further.

In the summary of her practice, the student related her contracting efforts in the first session. She followed her opening statement about the purpose of the group with a request for group members' ideas for the newletter. This is one example of *working from the production of the group members*.

The first session was exciting. It was filled with hope and expectations on the part of the worker as well as the members. The group expectation hung in the air. I had been talking and preparing for the group for several weeks and the newness of it was intriguing to the members. Most of the members had gotten to know me well enough to suspect that something different was happening, that this group would be different from other groups at the program.

In the beginning of the session, I explained to the group what I had in mind for the newsletter in order to clarify the purpose. I stated my purpose for the group. "As some of you already know, I had an idea to start a newsletter for this program. The newsletter would be created by all of you. You would write the articles, decide what went into them, how often it would be published and things like that. In other words, it would be your newsletter. I also thought of it as a way of helping the members of this program to get connected with each other and to keep each other informed as to what kinds of things happen around here. We could send copies to your friends and families to let them know what kinds of things you do here. I would also contribute my own ideas from time to time and be available to help members with any problems they might have. There will also be some other students and volunteers who have offered to help if any of you have trouble with writing. I'd like to hear from you now. Do you have any thoughts on this idea?"

In her analysis of the first session, the student realized that she had sensed ambivalence and doubt on the part of the members; however, she failed to reach for the underlying communications. She was unable, at that point, to *integrate her personal and professional selves* by using her feelings as a tool for exploring the potential negatives. In retrospect, it is easy to see how her own desire for a successful first session might have allowed her to ignore the signals rather than using the skill of "looking for trouble when everything is going your way." Her retrospective analysis also incorporates an *understanding of the group as a dynamic system.* This is evident as she shifts her view of the "deviant member" as an "enemy" to that of a group member sending a signal of underlying concerns.

Many members expressed interest and said it was a good idea, though I sensed some doubt on the part of the members. I had the vague sense they were just humoring me. Instead of confronting it directly I just went on, hoping in time they would become more invested. Had I confronted it then, it might have opened the discussion and raised some of the concerns and doubts they were feeling.

We decided a name for the newsletter and people volunteered for jobs. There was much debate about what to call the newsletter. Jim suggested "The Elite Newspaper of the East" as a possible title. He seemed very angry. I added his title to the rest of the titles to be voted upon and commented that I thought it was an interesting name. He did not respond and I went on collecting other titles. I realized I had not picked up the message he was sending me. I had missed the opportunity to address some of the anger he was feeling and I was not tuned into what was urgent to him at that moment. I was unable to set aside my own agenda. Had I picked up on his anger, I would have recognized that his feelings were representative of much of what the group was feeling. Fortunately for the group (and for me), this anger would surface again in later groups and help me break through the illusion of work that had formed.

Jim's sarcastic, self-deprecating title suggests the internalization of the oppressor as described in the oppression model. As the weeks passed, the group leader began to recognize that the behavior by some members in not doing their jobs represented a continuation of the unfinished business of the first session. She recognized that a general theme of disempowerment was emerging. She decided to *respond to these productions from the group members.* As the group members described being "treated like children," we can hear another signal of an indicator of oppression as they struggle to maintain their identity as adults. With the group given permission to explore the taboo area of its relationship to the system, Jim, the deviant member in the first session emerged as an internal leader.

During the fifth session, I noticed that many of the members were having difficulty concentrating and seemed completely disinterested in the group. I reached for what was happening. "What is going on today? Everyone seems to be having trouble focusing on the topic, and you all look bored and tired." Dan responded, "We all just went out for a long walk; we are tired." Richard added, "They keep us too busy around here, all we do is go to groups. They never leave us alone." I asked if anyone else felt this way and if they wanted to spend a few minutes talking about this.

Many members agreed with their comments and said they were feeling overwhelmed. I tried to validate their feelings by saying that sometimes there were a lot of groups to attend and then asked if they had ever spoken to the staff about this. Jim, the member who had been so angry in the first session, responded by saying that it did no good, the staff didn't care what they wanted, and that they were treated like children. I knew I had to be careful here. My natural inclination was to side with the group members. I had often been angered by the patronizing manner in which these men were treated. It would have been easy for me to have jumped on the bandwagon and started criticizing the hospital but I knew that would not be useful. I responded instead by reaching for his feelings. "It must feel pretty frustrating to be treated in this way. After all, you're not children, you're grown men." This opened the door for a lengthy discussion about how it felt to be a psychiatric patient and to lose so much control over one's life. I tried to bring the conversation back into focus by suggesting that the newsletter might be a forum the men could use to voice some of their concerns.

In the next excerpt, the principle of understanding the group as a dynamic system is illustrated again. Jim's comments represented the part of the group that felt oppressed and angry about the nature of the relationship with staff. Another set of feelings common to all members was fear of staff retribution and dependency on the system. This is expressed by Roland in the following excerpt. One can understand the ambivalence in the group as representing the internal ambivalence of each member. The inability of the group members to tolerate the stress, at this point, causes another member to take on the role of gatekeeper by changing the subject. In the same session we can observe the classic and maladaptive defense against depression–fight and flight.

> Roland, a member who I have always thought of as someone who was very ingratiating to the staff, eager and cooperative, fearful of making trouble, and generally considered a "good" patient, said, "Oh no, we couldn't do that; they would never let us print it. Besides, it's not really so bad around here. The staff are all nice and they treat us well." Another member seemed anxious after this interchange and completely changed the subject. Time was almost up so I said that if the group wanted to, we could continue talking about this the next time we met.

In the next excerpt, we see the group leader's growing confidence to trust her emotional responses as she deals directly with the indirect communications from staff who were concerned and threatened by the tone of the group discussions.

> The next session involved a field trip we had planned and, the session after that, the recreational therapist joined the

group. Apparently, the news had gotten out about our discussion. I told the staff I was encouraging the members to write about things that were meaningful to them and that at times this might involve an expression of criticism toward the hospital. They joked about how I was getting the patients all riled up. I sensed some suspicion beneath the humor. I asked if they thought this was a bad thing. This brought the issue out into the open and gave me the opportunity to speak with the staff about the patients' feelings.

In the session that follows, the leader once again responds to the indirect cues of the members and opens up a powerful area of discussion.

The next session we returned to the earlier topic. The members seemed distracted and uninterested. They were also having difficulties finishing their assignments. I asked them what was going on. Jimmy, a member who only occasionally attended, responded, "How do you expect us to do anything. I can't write, look at my hands." He held up his hands that were shaking visibly. "They keep us so medicated around here we can't even think straight." Jake agreed, "These doctors use us as guinea pigs. They try one medication after another. We are subjects in their experiments, they don't treat us like human beings."

Roland began to get nervous. "Yes, but we need to take our medications, it helps us. I'm ready for my next shot. I get too agitated if I don't get my shot." Jake responded, saying the medication did not help him, that it had ruined his life. He spoke of how he was not able to have a relationship with women or to live a normal life. He said, "Any member in this room will tell you that the medicine makes you impotent. How are you ever supposed to meet a girl or think about getting married." Several of the men nodded their heads in agreement. I said that must be very difficult for them and asked if they had ever let the doctors know about the problems they had with the medications. Jake again responded, "They don't care. If you refuse to take the medications, they will just lock you up." He went on to tell of how he had been forcibly locked up in the hospital.

Several other group members agreed, telling stories of how they had been locked in the seclusion room, been beaten by orderlies, or admitted to the hospital against their will. They said when they told someone, the doctors would say it was just their paranoia. Jake said that he was learning not to fight, that he was not a young man anymore. I empathized with the things that the group members had gone through and said it must be really difficult to always have someone questioning their reality. I then suggested that Jake might want to write about his experiences for the newsletter. I hoped to help empower them and to show them a way to have their concerns heard. Jake expressed ambivalence about doing this. I said I could understand his reservations and said if he wanted to he could take some time and think about it or that he could do it anonymously. This all proved to be more than Roland could stand.

Under his breath, but loudly enough for everyone to hear, he said "Communist!" I was taken aback by this expression of anger from Roland. I was also not sure who he was talking to. Jake responded angrily, "What did you call me?" Roland looked in his direction and said, louder this time, 'A communist. You're nothing but a communist. The doctors are just trying to help us. You're always going around trying to stir things up.' Jake was very angry at this. As a veteran, he considered this to be the worst insult. Jake responded to Roland, "I'm no communist, and don't you call me that. I have a right to say what I feel."

I was afraid the situation might escalate into violence, since Jake was extremely angry. (I also felt my maternal instincts surface.) I interjected, "Roland, it seems as if you see the situation in one way and Jake sees it from a different perspective. But I don't think it is useful for us to call each other names." I had intended to try to create a culture in which discussions of such matters were allowed and also one in which members respected and listened to one another. But, in rushing to Jake's defense, I was sending a message that I did not believe he could take care of himself and that he needed my protection. This was not a useful message to send to someone who already was feeling so oppressed. I might have done better if I had waited a little longer and allowed them to work things out themselves.

Roland apologized to Jake and said he was just a little "off" because he had not had his shot yet. Jake accepted this apology and the conversation returned to a discussion of an article someone was writing for the newsletter. The session ended with me encouraging the members to consider writing about their hospital experiences for the newsletter.

The interactional paradigm suggests that a group leader, in these circumstances, always has "two clients." Within the internal group system, the two clients are the individual and the group. The preceding practice excerpts have demonstrated the importance of the social worker's ability to simultaneously identify with each member of the group (Jim, Roland, Jake, etc.) and the group–as–a–whole. This mediating effort helps to break down the barriers between members, and by strengthening their bonding, reduces another indicator of oppression. In the external system that exists between the group and the environment, the group worker also has two clients, the first being the group and the second, the staff and the hospital system.

Over time, through careful work with both the group members and members of the staff system, the group leader was able to break through the negativity creating barriers between the two groups. Staff members overcame their concerns about the exposure of problems and anger in the system as they observed significant changes in the behavior of group members. The group leader continued to reach for the strength in the staff system, refusing to accept the behavior patterns that communicated a lack of caring. The worker's summary reflects her growing confidence in the process.

I can safely say the newsletter has become firmly established as a part of the program. I have noticed more staff members becoming invested in its continuation. There has been discussion of who will take over the project after I am gone. The director of the program requested a copy of the newsletter to be sent in with his semi-annual report, and another staff member included it in a presentation she was giving about the program. I have witnessed some change. The staff now relates in a slightly different manner toward the veterans. I notice some staff now saying "members" or "veterans" instead of patients. Many staff members appear to view the veterans in a new light. Several have expressed surprise over the talent that the men are exhibiting. There is also less fear and suspicion about what kinds of things I am doing with the group. We are still working on the issue of censorship. I continue to advocate for as little as possible in order to have the newsletter truly under the patients' control.

The group is still working on how much they want to express themselves in the newsletter. Many of the members still feel very disempowered and alienated, but they have been receiving a lot of positive reinforcement from the hospital community which has led to a tremendous boost in self-confidence and self-esteem. Some of the members of the newsletter group are working on submitting articles to a national journal that publishes work by disabled and hospitalized veterans. Others have expressed an interest in learning how to type so they can type the newsletter themselves. One member has decided to study for his G.E.D. This is truly an exciting process to watch.

This example illustrates how paradigm shifts in the psychology we use for assessment and in our models of the helping process can work together to dramatically alter our view of clients and our intervention strategies. The illustration also demonstrates the comfortable fit between the oppression psychology model and the interactional paradigm.

CONCLUSION: GROUP WORK'S CONTRIBUTION TO THE SHIFT IN THE SOCIAL WORK PARADIGM

It was suggested earlier that there are unique elements in group work that may account for its role in leading the profession through the paradigm shift described in this chapter. What are some of these elements?

First, the mutual aid model of group work, which incorporates a view of clients as having the inherent capacity to help each other, was an early precursor of the shift within the profession toward viewing clients from a strength perspective.

Second, as group work has emerged as an important tool for service for many oppressed and vulnerable populations (e.g., survivors of sexual abuse, persons with AIDS), it has contributed to the understanding of the long-term psycho-affective damages caused by persistent oppression. The comfortable fit between the interactional paradigm and the basic principles of the oppression model has served to reinforce their impact on both each other and the profession. The mutual aid process that I have described elsewhere (Shulman, 1992) as the "all-in-the-same-boat" and the "strength-in-numbers" phenomena, has helped social workers to see firsthand both the oppression-based sources of clients' problems as well as the healing powers of communal action.

Third, this same mutual aid process has helped social workers to rethink the basic medical paradigm that for so long has guided our work. In individual counseling, where control of the interview seems more completely vested in the hands of the helping professional, a linear view of the process may seem logical. In reality, even in individual interviews, control of the interview is still in the hands of the client who can choose whether or not to invest his or her heart, mind, and energy in the proceedings. In individual counseling, the illusion of an interview directed by the social worker is easier to maintain. In the less orderly processes of group work, where the strength-in-numbers phenomenon often allows the group members to seize control of the work, social workers have discovered how "letting go" can lead to their most effective sessions.

REFERENCES

Buhlan, H. A. *Frantz Fanon and the Psychology of Oppression*. New York: Plenum Press, 1985.

Germain, C. and A. Gitterman. *The Life Model of Social Work Practice*. New York: Columbia University Press, 1980.

Kuhn, T. *The Structure of Scientific Revolutions*. Chicago: University of Chicago Press, 1962.

Richmond, M. *Social Diagnosis*. New York: Russell Sage Foundation, 1918.

Shulman, L. *Identifying, Measuring and Teaching Helping Skills.* New York: Council on Social Work Education and the Canadian Association of Schools of Social Work, 1981.

Shulman, L. *Interactional Social Work Practice: Toward an Empirical Theory.* Itasca, Illinois: F. E. Peacock Publishers, Inc., 1991.

Shulman, L. *The Skills of Helping Individuals and Groups*, 3rd edition. Itasca, Illinois: F. E. Peacock Publishers, Inc., 1992.

Chapter 2

Making Joyful Noise: Presenting, Promoting, and Portraying Group Work to and for the Profession

Roselle Kurland
Robert Salmon

"Once more unto the breach, dear friends, once more; or close the wall up with our English dead!" (Shakespeare, *King Henry the Fifth*, act 3, scene 1, line 2). Does that sound familiar? Does the half-remembered line stir you a bit? It should as that surely was the intention of the author. Shakespeare gave Henry this line as the start of a powerful speech whose purpose was to rouse his vastly outnumbered forces to battle the French. His were the weapons of war of his time, as well as glorious language, and an appeal to courage.

The analogy to Henry is intentional. As we gather here today, we need to understand that we too are a vastly outnumbered force in a battle of a different kind. It *is* a battle–not bloody, but nevertheless intense–to preserve social work with groups as a viable part of social work practice today. The tools we use are not the symbolic primitive weapons of physical warfare. Ours are different. We need to use our knowledge of systems, of groups, and of individuals to preserve what we feel is important. These attributes, as well as organizational skills, and the " . . . use of humor and fun, playfulness along with planfulness in (our) practice approaches" (Middleman, 1990) are what we have to protect our method.

Plenary Presentation at the Fourteenth Annual Symposium of the Association for the Advancement of Social Work with Groups, October 1992, Atlanta, Georgia.

It needs protection. In a sobering research paper presented earlier this year, Martin Birnbaum and Charles Auerbach asked their audience to imagine a situation where social work students graduated without course work and field experience in work with individuals. The suggestion was inconceivable, but sadly it is often reality for group work. Most students are graduating without a group course and group work field experience and *are* likely to be practicing with groups. The irony is that work with groups is a major component of social work practice while graduate education has practically eliminated group work as a specialized area of study. (Birnbaum and Auerbach, 1992)

Two years ago, in a plenary address at the Twelfth Annual Symposium in Miami, Ruth R. Middleman delivered a call to action to those concerned with the place of group work in our profession. "Let us be noisy," she said.

Let us be watchdogs and whistle-blowers at omissions and misrepresentations concerning group work in our social work publications. Let us write interpretive statements about the breadth of group work, letters to the editors of journals, letters to the Educational Planning Commission of Council on Social Work Education and the Program Committee of the National Association of Social Workers (NASW), editorials for journals where we have influence. Let us accent an influence on the profession-at-large, sending our scholarship beyond the group journals. We must do our homework to prepare conceptual, scholarly, clarifying papers on social work with groups and provide interior views of our practice to others. (Middleman, 1990)

In this chapter, we build on Middleman's call to action to look at group work's current situation within the social work profession and consider strategies to present, promote, and portray group work to and for the profession.

It is almost sixty years since Wilbur Newstetter articulated the first definition of social group work (Newstetter, 1935), and yet many in our profession do not really understand or appreciate group work. That lack of understanding was also present in group work's preprofessional days before the 1930s when the majority of group workers worked in settlement houses, Y's, youth organizations, and playground and recreation departments (Wenocur and Reisch, 1989), *and* when the main focus of their work was on the well rather than the mentally ill. As Gertrude Wilson described it in 1937, group workers and caseworkers had little professional contact. She depicted a situation of mutual exclusiveness caused by indifference and latent antagonism characterized by only intermittent cooperation.

The problem of acceptance by other social work practitioners was felt by many group workers. The scorn exhibited toward "those workers who play with children," "run dances," "go camping," or "teach arts and crafts" is well remembered. In 1936 it was reported that the California Conference of Social Work seriously questioned whether group workers were social workers. Faculty members of the School of Social Service Administration of the University of Chicago minced no words in their exclusion of any study of an activity remotely connected with recreation. The general population of the country was still dominated by the "Protestant ethic" (Wilson, 1976).

Unfortunately, the lack of understanding of group work has not changed very much. Just three years ago, we invited ten outstanding alumni who had majored in group work at Hunter College School of Social Work to participate in a panel discussion. We asked them to identify what they thought were the most important things they had gained from their group work courses at Hunter and what they had not gotten, and what they wished they had because they realized now that they needed it. Almost to a person, what these alumni identified as needed was the ability to explain group work to others–to colleagues, supervisors, supervisees, professionals of other disciplines, and funding sources. They told of incidents and attitudes in their agencies that illustrated that group work was not well understood by professionals–social workers and others–with whom they came into contact. Said one graduate, a social worker in a hospital:

I was surprised to find that very few people know about group work, that there can be psychologists, psychiatrists, and social workers, too, who just think that social group work is casework in a group. You just throw the group together and talk to each person, and you control everything, and then that's fine, you have started a group. . . . The other thing that I found surprising is how much group work is looked down upon. It's not acknowledged as an actual training with its own theories and its own skills. . . . It has been a struggle for me to communicate to other disciplines that social workers *do* know something about running groups. (Cavrell-Epstein, 1989)

Another graduate, a social worker in a community mental health clinic, lamented that other social workers in his agency seemed to have little understanding of or appreciation for work with groups. "They do not really think that the work that I do with clients is important," he said. "It's individual therapy that they view as the real work, not group work" (Munoz, 1989). And still another graduate, a director of a small agency working with youth, said she struggled to explain group work to representatives of foundations and other funding sources. "When funders make a site visit and come into a room and see the kids working on a project together and maybe it seems chaotic, how do you explain that what's going on is important, that there's more to it than meets the eye?" she asked (Lyons, 1989).

Underlying the difficulty in explaining group work to others in social work, we believe, is a lack of respect that many, though certainly not all, in our profession hold toward group work. That lack of respect is difficult to combat, for often it is not expressed directly. Group work is *said* to be respected, but beneath the surface lurks attitudes that assert: "If you know how to work with individuals, then you can work with a group for group work is simply casework multiplied," or "Group work is superficial. It's only in individual work where there is true depth," or "Activities, so often used by group workers, aren't really helpful. The psychological insights that stem from discussion of problems are what matter."

We have faced these attitudes toward group work throughout our history. Group work's use of activities, for instance, has been causing professional discomfort for sixty years or more. The early group workers who moved into social work from recreation and leisure-time programs were viewed with skepticism then and questions about whether they really were social workers (Middleman, 1982). For many social workers, that is not so different today.

> After much "lobbying" on her part a second-year social work student, whose placement was at a large state hospital for the mentally ill, convinced the director of in-patient services to allow her to form and lead a singing group. Her supervisor's attitude toward her work with the singing group was made quite evident when she told the student, "Do not bother to write process recordings on the singing group. We don't have to talk much about that group. Just do process for your therapy group."

Many in social work, even today, do not understand or appreciate the value of activity in group work practice. They are much more at ease with and accord higher status and legitimacy to group work practice that uses words exclusively. Helen Harris Perlman, reviewing changes in the first decade of the NASW, 1955-1965, sounded almost relieved when she wrote about group work.

> It has burst the too narrow seams of its basketball uniform and arts-and-crafts smocks; increasingly it appears in the contrasting symbolic garments that bespeak the poles of its present scope—the authority-cool white coats of hospital and clinical personnel and the play-it-cool windbreaker of the street-corner gang worker . . . group work is increasingly involved with the persons, places, problems and even some of the processes that not too long ago were assumed to 'belong' to case work. (Perlman, 1965)

Greatly contributing to the misconceptions that social workers have about group work and the need to explain our method to our colleagues in social work is the current state of graduate social work education. The paucity of curriculum content on work with groups and the causes of that vacuum have been described in papers and plenary addresses at past symposia (Birnbaum, 1990; Middleman, 1990; Parry, 1991).

These presentations have made us aware that, from the 1960s on, the CSWE moved toward curriculum standards that required schools of social work to emphasize the *generic* in social work practice. The move was intended to define more sharply social work's identity as one profession. That effort, however, has been a disaster for group work. Left out and rapidly disappearing from our profession are the *specific* beliefs, knowledge, and skills that are the hallmark of group work.

Because group workers were always a small minority of social work faculty, generic practice courses, by necessity, were taught largely by persons whose expertise was in work with individuals and who had little or no social group work experience. The emphasis in such courses was on either work with individuals or on a kind of group work that focuses on individual group members to the neglect of the group, or on the individual and the psychological to the neglect of the social.

Given the growing neglect of group work in graduate social work education for close to three decades, it is no wonder that our graduates cry out that their colleagues do not understand, appreciate, or respect group work. It is no wonder that they have difficulty explaining it.

So where do we go from here? What are the implications for action of group work's current situation? What do we need to do to present, promote, and portray group work to and for the profession? How can we go about making joyful noise? We recommend seven directions that our efforts must take.

First, we ourselves must get better at articulating the value and uniqueness of group work's approach to (and emphasis in) working with people. The humanistic views that undergird our work, the need of people for acceptance, for belonging, and for group membership, the quest for social justice and for social change, for consciousness-raising and empowerment—all of these have been spoken and written about with conviction and eloquence by participants in past symposia* and all are vital to an identification of group work's

---

*See, for example, Urania Glassman and Len Kates, *Group Work: A Humanistic Approach*, Sage Publications, 1990; Hans Falck, *Social Work: The Membership Perspective*, New York: Springer Publishing Company, 1988; Margot Breton, "Learning From Social Group Work Traditions," *Proceedings*, 11th Annual Symposium on Social Work With Groups, Montreal, 1989.

uniqueness and importance.What remains pivotal, as well, to an articulation of the uniqueness and specialness of group work is the concept of mutual aid, described first by Peter Kropotkin (1914) and made central to group work by William Schwartz (1971). The process of mutual aid really is unique to social group work. We need to get better at identifying its importance and depicting what mutual aid looks like in group work practice.

In a previous publication (Kurland and Salmon, 1992), the authors attempted to do this by discussing the major differences between group work and casework in a group. In fact, *casework in a group* can be defined as practice that does not maximize mutual aid among group members. Casework in a group is mutual aid-less! It can be seen when a worker views each member only as an individual and applies individual personality theories and dynamics without appreciating or understanding the impact of such group concepts as size, roles, norms, communication patterns, member interaction and influence, and group stages, to name but a few. Similarly, casework in a group is being practiced when a worker allots time to each individual group member, in turn, to talk about progress on issues of concern or when a worker allots time in round-robin fashion and does not maximize group interaction.

Group work, on the other hand, can be defined as a process where mutual aid is central and maximized. In such group work practice, the situation, problem, or need of one group member provides an opportunity for *all* in the group to examine their own situations, problems, or needs as they draw upon their own experiences to respond to their fellow members. Merely jumping in to give advice to another member is *not* group work. In fact, it is the quality of the *mutual* aid process that occurs in a group that is central in distinguishing social group work practice from other group efforts. We need to talk about the mutual aid process more, and more clearly, as we attempt to describe group work to others.

Second, we need to develop data to support our claim that the lack of group work education and training matters. The reality that many groups are being led today by workers untrained in social group work practice has been identified previously as problematic (Birnbaum, Middleman, and Huber, 1989). But we need to do more than bemoan that fact. We need to be able to identify what difference that makes. We need evidence.

A recently completed research study by Dominique Moyse Steinberg (1992) is an important step in providing some of the evidence we need. Steinberg interviewed some 30 social workers who were working with groups, half of whom had substantial graduate social work education in group work and half of whom had minimal or no group work education or training. She spoke with them in depth about their practice with groups and found important differences between those with group work education and those without it.

There were differences in the way these workers conceptualized the group, exercised control, and viewed their role and their use of self. Those without education in group work tended to see the group as a place for individual change within a supportive environment. They tended to play a central role throughout the group's life, to direct many of their interventions to individual group members, and to assume a great deal of control. Those with group work education expected the group members to integrally affect and effect the shape and movement of the group. They saw group purpose as central. They tended to direct many of their interventions and expectations to the group as a whole and to be aware of the impact the stages of group development had over time on their role and their use of themselves.

Especially important were differences regarding conflict held by these workers. While those with group work education expected conflict to occur as a natural result of group life and viewed conflict as opportunity for important work in the group, those without education in group work tended to regard conflict as an intrusion into the group's affairs, an unwelcome interruption, a threat to the group, and a hurdle that needed to be quickly resolved so that the group could move on.

Steinberg's findings are important. They tell us that group work education really does matter and that who leads a group makes a difference in the quality of professional practice. They provide us with the kind of evidence that we need to argue for greater attention to group work in social work education and agency supervision and training. They provide much direction for future efforts and research. We need more such work to use in our attempts to substantiate the importance of group work education.

Third, we need to present both our articulation of group work's uniqueness and importance and our evidence that group work education and training make a difference to a wide range of people–to students and supervisees, to colleagues, to agency supervisors and administrators, to social work faculty members, to deans and directors of schools of social work, to CSWE, to NASW.

Our efforts to establish group work's place in both education and practice need to go in two directions simultaneously. From the bottom up, our students, supervisees, and colleagues in agencies and on faculties might well be helped to become ambassadors, even missionaries perhaps, for the practice and teaching of group work where it is needed. From the top down, our deans and administrators, and our national organizations need to be helped to see that group work is endangered. They must be held accountable for ensuring that social group work is not allowed to disappear.

The efforts of AASWG and many of its members to influence CSWE's curriculum policy statements, establish a presence on its policy-making boards, and open lines of communication and collaboration with NASW certainly are steps in this direction. We must continue to make our presence known with ever-increasing vigor and be both reactive and proactive as we engage with our national social work organizations.

Fourth, we, ourselves, must become involved in agency training, consultation, and supervision. We need to use our beliefs and passion about the importance of group work, our knowledge and our skills to enhance workers' understanding, appreciation, and respect for groups and group work practice, and to improve their skill in group leadership.

We need to go out of our way to be responsive to calls for help from agencies and practitioners who are interested in work with groups.

Five years ago at the tenth annual symposium in Baltimore, I was approached by two young individuals from Iowa whom I did not know. Would I be willing to supervise them around their work with groups of teenagers who had been sexually abused, they wanted to know. They had tried to obtain supervision from staff at the agency where they were leading groups, as well as from professionals outside the agency, but were unable to find anyone with expertise in social group work. They had even looked for courses on group work that they might take. To put it mildly, I was surprised at their request. How would this work, I wanted to know. They suggested telephone supervision once a month. I had my doubts. But their earnestness, the initiative they took in approaching me, their commitment to their work, and their desire for help were impossible to disregard.

I agreed and thus began one of the most unusual and rewarding professional relationships I have experienced. We spoke on the phone for an hour or more once a month for over a year until their work with teens ended. Each month we had to make sure we had the time straight for our calls–"O.K., seven o'clock your time, that's eight o'clock my time." The conversations were fun and exciting. They directed our conversations with questions and concerns that they had and the situations they described. Often, they challenged my responses– "But why are you suggesting that? Could you say more about what you mean?"–and made *me* really think. Our common interest in the work united us even when we hardly knew each other and could not even talk face-to-face. We all benefited. (Kurland, 1992)

There is a real thirst for knowledge about groups out there and we need to respond to it in creative ways. We need to share our expertise in work with groups, to make it available to others.

One special group with which we need to work is field instructors to help them supervise students around work with groups. Another might be faculty members who want to expand their knowledge. Our efforts need to be aimed to help both agency staff and faculty understand that it is in their interest and that of their clients and students to move to the inclusion and/or expansion of groups (Kurland, Getzel, and Salmon, 1986).

Fifth, we need to continue to talk to ourselves. Doing so strengthens our ability to then go out and talk to others. At these symposia, in the local chapters of AASWG, and through the journal, *Social Work with Groups*, we find our voice and our song and revitalize and energize ourselves.

If history is instructive, then we can learn from the past that we need a place of our own within a social work profession where work with individuals predominates. A place where we can share our ideas, and practice with others with similar interests and experiences. The formation of the AASWG in 1979 came as a response to such a need, just as in 1946 group workers felt it was necessary to form their own organization, the American Association of Group Workers (Wenocur and Reisch, 1989).

Sixth, we need to develop our scholarship and write and speak about our work in special group work forums such as the journal *Social Work with Groups*, these symposia, and the group work section of CSWE's annual program meeting. Additionally, we must also present our work in the forums of our profession throughout its many journals and conferences.

> Last spring we submitted an abstract for a paper we wished to present at the annual program meeting of CSWE. We purposely did *not* submit it as part of the specialized group work section, for we wanted to speak to a wider audience. Much to our surprise, we received a call from one of the professional staff at the Council. Wanting to be helpful, she asked whether we had made a mistake. Since the words "group work" were in the abstract's title, she wondered whether we meant to submit it to the special group work section. When we told her that no mistake had been made, she said that it certainly was possible to consider our abstract a general submission.

We do ourselves a disservice when we talk *only* to each other. We need to present our ideas and our work to a diverse social work audience if that work is to have impact and influence. We cannot allow others to isolate our work and our ideas and we cannot isolate ourselves.

Too often, our presentations and papers just describe our work with groups. Though description of our work is important, it is not enough. Our scholarship needs to bring together the doing and the thinking of group work practice. Descriptions of practice need to be examined conceptually, critically, analytically. Presentations of work with groups will be strengthened and made more useful if description is linked to theory. In an editorial in *Social Work with Groups*, the editors (Roselle Kurland and Andrew Malekoff, 1992) discuss the kinds of articles they would like to see submitted to the journal. They note, "In articles that portray practice through the presentation of descriptive vignettes and examples, the rationale that underpins the practice, the thinking behind it, and the implications for future practice with groups are crucial elements" (Kurland and Malekoff, 1992).

Seventh, we need to begin to encourage and develop the scholars and teachers of group work's future. When we encounter workers with interest in and passion for work with groups, we should ask whether they have considered teaching, be it on a full-time basis or as adjunct instructors. We need to make ourselves available as mentors for such persons and support their efforts to engage in the teaching and training of new social workers. Those with conviction about and commitment to group work need to become a force and a presence on social work faculties. To do so, they will need to develop well-rounded expertise in areas beyond group work. Then, as they teach courses, such as human behavior, research, and practice and policy, in addition to specialized courses in group work, they will bring their sensitivity and understanding of groups and group work practice to those courses. They will have an impact.

The actions that we are recommending to present, promote, and portray group work are really not so very new. There are no miraculous elixirs; hard work is required of us. We have tried to be very practical and quite specific in delineating what we must do. In summary, we propose seven areas on which to focus our energy.

- We need to get better at articulating the value and uniqueness of group work.
- We need to develop hard evidence to demonstrate that the paucity of group work education and training is a problem.
- We need to widely disseminate both our articulation and our evidence.
- We need to get involved in agency training, consultation, and supervision.

- We need to continue to talk to ourselves.
- We need to develop our scholarship and write and speak about our work in specialized group work forums as well as in the wider forums of the social work profession.
- We need to encourage and develop the scholars and teachers of group work's future.

Social group work is a very positive and optimistic way of working with people. It is truly empowering. It is truly affirming of people's strengths. It is a fact that the very act of forming a group is a statement of belief in people's strengths, a statement of belief that everyone has something to give to others. In today's troubled world, real group work is needed more than ever. We cannot let it disappear. We truly must make joyful noise.

REFERENCES

Birnbaum, Martin. (1990, October). "Group Work, the Spotted Owl: An Endangered Species in Social Work Education." Presented at the 12th annual Symposium on Social Work with Groups, Miami, Florida.

Birnbaum, Martin, Middleman, Ruth, and Huber, Ruth. (1989). "Where Social Workers Obtain Their Knowledge Base in Group Work." Presented at the Annual Meeting of NASW.

Birnbaum, Martin and Auerbach, Charles. (1992, March). "Group Work in Graduate Social Work Education–The Price of Neglect." Presented at the Council on Social Work Education Annual Program meeting, Kansas City, Kansas.

Breton, Margot. (1989, October). "Learning from Social Group Work Traditions." Proceedings of the Eleventh Annual Symposium on Social Work with Groups, Montreal, Canada.

Cavrell-Epstein, Dawn. (1989). Panel discussion. Hunter College School of Social Work, New York, New York, November 9.

Falck, Hans. (1988). *Social Work: The Membership Perspective*. New York: Springer Publishing Company.

Glassman, Urania and Kates, Len. (1990). *Group Work: A Humanistic Approach*. Sage Publications, Inc., Newbury Park, CA.

Kropotkin, Peter. (1914). *Mutual Aid: A Factor of Evolution*. Reissued in 1989 by Black Rose Books: Montreal, Canada.

Kurland, Roselle. (1992, September). Personal statement to class at Hunter College School of Social Work.

Kurland, Roselle, Getzel, George, and Salmon, Robert. (1986). "Sowing Groups in Infertile Fields: Curriculum and Other Strategies to Overcome Resistance to the Formation of New Groups." In *Innovations in Social Work: Feedback From Practice to Theory*, Marvin Parnes (Ed.). New York: The Haworth Press.

Kurland, Roselle and Malekoff, Andrew. (1992). Editorial. *Social Work with Groups*, Vol. 15, No. 4, pp. 1-2.

Kurland, Roselle and Salmon, Robert. (1992). "Group Work vs. Casework in a Group: Principles and Implications for Teaching and Practice." *Social Work with Groups*, Vol. 15, No. 4, pp. 3-14.

Lyons, Eileen. (1989). Panel discussion. Hunter College School of Social Work, New York, New York, November 9.

Middleman, Ruth. (1982). *The Non-Verbal Method in Working with Groups*, enlarged edition. Hebron, CT: Practitioners' Press.

Middleman, Ruth. (1990, October). "Group Work and the Heimlich Maneuver: Unchoking Social Work Education." Plenary Address, 12th Annual Symposium on Social Work with Groups, Miami, Florida.

Munoz, Manuel. (1989). Panel discussion. Hunter College School of Social Work, New York, New York, November 9.

Newstetter, Wilbur. (1935). "What is Social Group Work?" *Proceedings of the National Conference of Social Work*, pp. 291-299. New York: National Conference of Social Work.

Parry, Joan. (1991, October). Plenary Address, 13th Annual Symposium on Social Work With Groups, Akron, Ohio.

Perlman, Helen Harris. (1965). "Social Work Method: A Review of the Past Decade." *Social Work*, Vol. X, No. 4.

Schwartz, William and Zalba, Serapio. (1971) *The Practice of Group Work*. New York: Columbia University Press.

Shakespeare, William. *King Henry the Fifth*, III, I, 2.

Steinberg, Dominique Moyse. (1992). *The Impact of Group Work Education on Social Work Practitioners' Work with Groups*. Doctoral dissertation, City University of New York, New York.

Wenocur, Stanley and Reisch, Michael. (1989). *From Charity to Enterprise: The Development of Social Work in a Market Economy*. Urbana: University of Illinois Press.

Wilson, Gertrude. (1976). "From Practice to Theory: A Personalized History." In *Theories of Social Work with Groups*. Robert Roberts and Helen Northen (Eds.). New York: Columbia University Press.

Chapter 3

AIDS and Group Work:
Looking into the Second Decade
of the Pandemic

George S. Getzel

It is not speculative to indicate that the end of the twentieth century will be associated with the mounting specter of the worldwide AIDS pandemic–estimated to reach a cumulative toll of 40 million people in the next eight years (Altman, 1991). The burden of grief in cities such as New York, San Francisco, Los Angeles, and Newark cannot humanly be encompassed. How do you begin to absorb the reality of thousands of youngsters orphaned after both parents have died of AIDS in New York City (Narvarro, 1990) and the 10 million children throughout the world estimated to die by the year 2000 ("Children AIDS cases are reported to rise," 1990)?

As with incidents of mass deaths from war, natural disasters, and epidemics, the inevitable response to AIDS has been the unrelenting denial of the actual magnitude of the problem (Camus, 1952; Shilts, 1988; Kramer, 1989). No one wants to think about the number of people dead and dying, or the consequences of their deaths on surviving kin, friends, and neighbors. By analogy, it took some 40 years after the Nazi Holocaust before survivors were recognized as victims of an unimaginable mass slaughter. Survivors of mass death must contend with the disbelief of those shielded from the direct experience of their tragedies. Denial may falter when the human face of massive cumulative death can be depicted in a manner that portrays it on a scale that allows for some tolerance of an otherwise incomprehensible reality (Getzel and Masters, 1984; Getzel and Mahony, 1990).

For group workers the denial of tragedy and the re-experiencing of a past painful event on a more manageable scale is a familiar phenomenon in the small-group context. Groups allow their memberships the security and the comfort to face ultimate boundary issues of loss and death. This may explain the widespread use of groups to support people with AIDS (PWAs), their loved ones and those volunteers and professionals who work with PWAs (Gambe and Getzel, 1989; Rounds, Galinsky, and Stevens, 1991; Lopez and Getzel, 1986). In the group context, AIDS, which combines themes of illness, death, and oppression, is more related in a comprehensible and concrete manner to the public issues of social ostracism and the abrogation of human rights that obstructs access to needed resources.

OBJECTIVES

This chapter will use the author's direct experience caring for a PWA as a way of exploring the special demands on persons who face the consequences of AIDS in their daily living and in their general outlook toward the world. The central issues addressed in small groups of PWAs and their caregivers will be identified as well as the special benefits that group work offers to these populations. The theoretical nature of practice with PWAs will be examined for its broad implications for group work in the coming decade. Areas for future group work development during the AIDS pandemic will be specified.

PERSONAL PERSPECTIVE

In an effort to bring the human face of AIDS alive, I want to recount some personal experiences that occurred within a 15-hour period. I strongly believe that the events that follow contain the essential elements of what the AIDS epidemic has taught me and will regrettably continue to teach me. Finally, I also think that the AIDS epidemic makes a persuasive argument for the healing powers of groups.

AN UNCERTAIN CONDITION

On an afternoon last October my phone rang: it was a nurse telling me that my friend Kevin, a PWA, was seriously ill in his doctor's office. She asked if I could immediately come to be with him. I had assumed significant responsibility for Kevin's care after he was diagnosed with AIDS.

After being given an injection in his doctor's office, Kevin went into shock; his fingertips had turned purple; he spiked a fever of over 104°; and he had become mentally confused. His doctor would not allow him go home alone; and if Kevin's condition continued to worsen, he would have to go to the emergency room of the hospital. The prospect of that dreadful scenario brought to mind a Kafkaesque episode that Kevin and I shared a year earlier: we waited four and a half days in the emergency room before getting a bed in the hospital. Feelings of depression and dread surged back.

Rushing to Kevin, never knowing when or where I would be needed, had become a way of life. Despite serial crises, we continued to try to live as normally as possible, yet always harboring a sense of an imminent reversal of bodily and mental well-being. A life full of people with AIDS and a great deal of knowledge did not wholly help us maintain a balanced emotional response to the hurts, the indignities, and the dislocations occasioned by the unrelenting downward trajectory of Kevin's health. Candor and generally open communications did, however, help us face the accelerating decline of Kevin's functional capacity and the appearance of dementia symptoms.

Despite all my fears and apprehensions, being there for him was always comforting; that was the case when I saw him resting in the examining room that afternoon. My panic and numbness vanished. I was again present to bear witness to his suffering, find a way to comfort him, and be comforted by him. Kevin looked relieved when I finally arrived. He wept at the prospect of going back to the emergency room and held my hand.

When I looked at him that afternoon, I became painfully aware of the stark physical changes that he had undergone—especially the loss of weight made obvious by the cavernous spaces that surrounded his still-beautiful blue eyes. In my reverie, I recalled a conversation that we recently had about the blank stare that so many PWAs exhibit as they approach death, a far-off, disconnected gaze. Painfully, I saw that look in Kevin.

Also that afternoon, I was absorbed in thinking about the delicate connection between a sense of well-being and the bodily substrata that can change so dramatically. A glimpse of our human finiteness was inescapable.

After an hour Kevin's temperature did not rise further. Through some splendid collusion with his physician, Kevin was sent home. After we arrived at the apartment, his mood became positively optimistic: we discussed a trip to the Southwest. Kevin said I looked exhausted and that I should go home; he would call me if anything came up. It was hard leaving him, but I was exhausted. I took the subway home.

As I approached my subway stop, I closed my eyes, only to feel a cold circle of metal against my temple. My eyes opened to see a young man in a hooded sweat shirt and dark glasses. He told me if I gave him all my money, nothing would happen to me. I fumbled and absent-mindedly found dollar bills in my jacket and wallet which seemed to bemuse him. I said to myself that it had not been a bad life; that I had accomplished a great deal. If my life were to end now, it would be difficult for my spouse and children, but they would survive. I was concerned that my sudden death would over-whelm Kevin, but what was I to do? In this state of mind, I was chagrined at my objectivity, which was strange and fascinating under the circumstances.

As quickly as the young man appeared before my open eyes, he disappeared, slipping through the subway car's closing doors, one stop from my destination. I was left feeling as if it was an odd dream.

CRISIS SITUATION

I felt peculiarly prepared for the event of that evening. I thought about the life that Kevin had led since becoming diagnosed with AIDS. I finally decided what had happened to me was not a dream while I recounted my story in detail to the police who, although sympathetic, convinced me that my tale was routine. Later that evening my family heard my story with alarm.

Sleep was somehow restful, which brings me to the third and final event of those hours. The next morning I went to work on the subway through the Upper West Side of Manhattan. Toward the end of my trip as the train left a subway station, I heard a scream, "Oh my God!" The subway car seemed to make a gentle leap that occasioned a scraping noise, a spray of sparks, and the smell of rancid fumes. Pandemonium broke out as some of the younger passengers thought the car was about to explode. Powerful odors overwhelmed and choked me. I was quickly convinced that the train had run over a person who apparently jumped in front of the motor-man's car.

While the final event of that day is not an ordinary aspect of my travels in the City, I was struck by my attitude toward this tragic occurrence. Where were my emotional agitation and my revulsion? Was I considering a suicidal death to be commonplace?

Clearly, after these 15 hours I could use a support group to handle the cumulative trauma. Fortunately, there was such a group for me. Also, working with groups of people with AIDS and their caregivers has provided me with both understanding and knowledge to assist me in reaching a point of emotional equilibrium, and in facing more closely the questions of death and dying. Upon reflection, it is the experiences of knowing PWAs that has contributed significantly to whatever wisdom and forbearance I have to manage serial trauma. I am forever grateful that PWAs have been a part of my life, in many cases far too briefly.

IDENTITY CONCERNS

I believe that the inner reality of death shifted for me, in large part, due to the experiences of knowing so many young people, including friends, who have died in rapid succession. After seeing PWAs undergo series of elongated, debilitating, and humiliating health reverses, I now see death as relief from an unacceptable condition. Two of my closest friends asked my "permission" to die, and if it was acceptable to bid me farewell. During these extraordinary moments before their approaching deaths, they and I knew, however difficult the words were to say, death was absolutely OK. Moreover, it was a biological and human necessity not to have a slavish attachment to physiological life, to do so was to demean the importance of living. The irony of discussing "when enough was enough" with dying friends was that they presented eloquent statements of their enduring human identity.

THEORETICAL PERSPECTIVE

Erikson (1964) in this respect writes that, "Any span of the cycle lived without vigorous meaning, at the beginning, in the middle, or at the end, endangers the sense of life and the meaning of death in all whose life stages are intertwined. . . . Individuality here finds its ultimate test, namely, man's existence at the entrance to that valley which he must cross alone" (p. 133).

Talking about rational suicide, the saving of pills with the intention of accomplishing that end, and even the preparing of others for an eventual planned death are common subjects for PWAs. I believe such discussions reflect efforts to foster a cognitive perspective and a value stance that would otherwise elude them.

Identity or the presence of a personal ego provides the central anchor that all human beings need to maintain an abiding sense of individuality without feeling fractionated or divisible into a nameless mass of other human creatures. Erikson (1964) notes that all human beings must protect themselves through maintaining a "sense of wholeness, a sense of centrality in time and space, and a sense of freedom of choice" (p. 148-149), through secret delusions and collective illusions maintained by the current and internalized interpersonal relationships. Any life-threatening disease or chronically disabling condition has the potential to play havoc with an individual's ego integrity or identity. AIDS, with its high-profile social stigma, severely threatens personal identity by weakening the interpersonal resources available to grapple with serial crises.

RITES OF PASSAGE

Another significant aspect of the experience of AIDS is the moving from one definition of self to another imbued with apparent and subtle references to an emerging identity linked to AIDS. I recalled that after Kevin was diagnosed with AIDS, he said that he just had his bar mitzvah. For him, diagnosis was a predictable rite of passage as it had been for so many of his gay friends. Beyond the dark humor of Kevin's characterization, was his effort to regularize, to order the disorderly out-of-control disease entity that now entered his life.

Many people with AIDS resist an identity suffused with meanings related to AIDS in an effort not to allow it to dominate their everyday living. To the extent that this form of denial abets coping with the issues of getting through the demands of daily living, it should not be challenged by kin, friends, and professionals. Alongside the support of positive denial should be a willingness to address in an honest and straightforward manner the real-life consequences of HIV/AIDS. Although we all should protest the injustices and human rights dangers affecting PWAs, the question of assuming a new identity dictated by the progress of the disease as well as societal bigotry remains a vital concern.

The pervasive presence of AIDS-related fears and obsessions in society cannot be underestimated. For example, a few years ago when I lost a great deal of weight I found myself confronted by several friends who asked me if I now had an AIDS diagnosis. I told them that I appreciated their concern, but I did not have AIDS to the best of my knowledge. One colleague noted afterward to a friend in common that I really had AIDS and just was covering it up. From a societal perspective, this persistent colleague was partially correct, my association with the issue of HIV/AIDS and PWAs gives me an AIDS identity and who am I to refute it?

RATIONALE FOR GROUPS

Group work addresses AIDS as: (1) an uncertain, life-threatening condition reminding us of our human finitude that evokes; (2) continuous crisis situations that; and (3) severely challenge the ego identities of affected people. The use of groups for PWAs, caring kin, and others is posited to create the conditions by which members can address the cognitive, emotional, and action requirements necessary to confront these challenges that may not be as successfully handled through dyadic exchanges or even family treatment (Getzel, 1991a).

From evidence in groups of people with AIDS and their caregivers, social isolation is frequently mentioned as one of the most disturbing aspects of dealing with AIDS. Feelings of isolation and estrangement from others reflect the disengagement of PWAs after having experienced rejection or anticipated rejection from kin, friends, colleagues, employers and others, in no small part due to the stigma that is still attached to HIV infection and an AIDS diagnosis (Christ, Weiner, and Moynihan, 1986; Lopez and Getzel, 1984). Quite typically, the first sessions of a group of persons affected by HIV or AIDS consists of members telling "war stories" of sorts. These describe the serial rejections and abandonment by others as word of their AIDS diagnosis became known. Expressing rage and hurt is frustrated when group members believe there is no way they can adequately give form to the depth of what they are feeling. It is the therapeutic factor of universalization, long recognized as a potent benefit of group experiences (Yalom, 1984) that provides the precondition for the group process to assist the membership's examination of the consequences of the disease.

The almost immediate sense of relief experienced in the early sessions of groups is remarkable. Group workers should not mistake this phenomenon as representing the diminished importance of their roles in AIDS support groups. Group workers should appreciate the power of these groups to provide a forum to discuss the trials and tribulations of interpreting their situations to family members, friends, and professionals involved in their care.

The significance of being able to open up otherwise unspeakable feelings and thoughts is of utmost importance. These early explorations in groups entail discussions of being diagnosed with HIV/AIDS and initial hospitalizations that become the building blocks for testing trust within the group. This group process presages confrontations with significant others who are not fully accepting or knowledgeable about their health condition.

To the extent group workers are unable to listen to the underlying messages encoded in the routine problem solving that occurs in PWA and caregiver support groups, they will support members in unconsciously evading the issue of early death. The so-called "D" word may be momentarily mentioned in the group only to create a consensus that is not appropriate, because the group should only be used for the discussion of living successfully with AIDS. Implicit in this wish-laden formulation is that dying is failure, and speaking about it will magically lead to death. Amazingly, these shared illusions can be quite sturdy and formidable, that is, until a member has a near-death experience or dies.

LIFE CYCLE RE-ENACTMENT

The particular strength of the group experience lies in the possibility of members symbolically engaging in a life cycle re-enactment, in a period of months that families typically undergo over generations. It is the reactions of group members to this re-enactment that prepare them as individuals for the mortal consequences of AIDS.

Death can be understood realistically in a twofold perspective—of the life that one is leaving and the process of letting go of that life. Erikson (1964) has called that capacity, "wisdom . . . detached concern with life itself, in the face of death itself" (p. 133).

The group provides a secure environment to develop attachment to others, and if fate determines that you will lose group members, you may let go of them with the enhanced recognition of what their parting has taught you. Despite the pain and rage that many members express about the death of their peers, they will freely acknowledge what the gift of other group members' lives has given them (Getzel, 1991b). On one occasion, group members shared with each other that the extended and heroic dying of one member served as a source of inspiration. As one member said, "I don't know if I could have Robert's courage, but it helps me know that he is struggling with so much dignity. He is also concerned about us after he has become blind and paralyzed." A long silence followed with some men weeping that Robert would no longer be at meetings. He was not forgotten.

The task of the group worker is to assist the members to neither merge with expressions of denial of the realistic burdens of illness nor wallow in a morbid, clawing preoccupation with dying. The group provides an arena for the playing out of members' more extreme reactions to AIDS as a disease of loss, separation, and death. The group present models of acceptance of finite conditions and problem solving in the here-and-now.

LEGACY AND IDENTITY

The urge for affirmation of an identity in the face of bodily dissolution and for the creation of a legacy as a way of being remembered after death creates strong ambivalence within groups of PWAs. Lingering doubts of self-worth related to the incorporation of past negative valuations emerge as PWAs more realistically face the question of personal mortality. In a complementary fashion, caregivers struggle with wishes that the burdens of caregiving be more fully appreciated by PWAs and others; also that their burdens be over for themselves and their very sick loved ones. The thought that very sick PWAs might be better off dead evokes agitated periods of guilt; caregivers, as they are able to directly express these thoughts in the group, come through a vital process of greater acceptance and personal validation of their often heroic efforts and self-denial. For caregivers who were also sexual partners of dying PWAs, their own sense of vulnerability is magnified through closely observing the physical decline of loved ones because a vital subject is legitimated through group discussion. What would be a taboo can be addressed, and emotional understanding occurs, which better prepares group members to handle their approaching bereavement.

THE FUTURE

We are now in the second decade of the AIDS pandemic, which in some ways is "Back to the Future." Despite the fact that women, children, adolescents, people of color, and heterosexually oriented persons are being HIV infected and diagnosed with AIDS in larger numbers than ever before, the federal government has not become significantly more responsive to the needs of PWAs. Clearly, lessons painfully learned in the last decade are not being exploited to save lives now. Although it may be 1992, in some respects it feels like 1982. The use of groups and peer teaching about safer sex and AIDS must be extended to schools, churches, single bars, or wherever they can provide the social skills and information to prevent the spread of the HIV infection.

Groups have given "safe harbor" to persons directly affected by HIV and AIDS, and have also been a crucial source of support to social workers and others providing services to people. The fiction of "autonomous practice" is especially ludicrous for professionals working with PWAs who must face complicated and difficult personal reactions, value dilemmas, and ethical issues.

From the point of view of the development of group work practice, knowledge gained from working with PWAs provides an opportunity to fill a significant gap in theory about how to work with persons with a terminal illness.

Questions of the quality of life of very ill persons and decision making about the extent of care patients desire have taken on increased importance. Group workers have an important role in helping PWAs and their caregivers receive the support necessary to think and understand the implications of quality-of-life decisions that they are being forced to address.

The use of groups for PWAs and others affected by the AIDS pandemic is becoming even more widespread. Every social agency with people with AIDS must now give consideration to the formation of support groups for persons affected including staff support groups, as the pandemic expands in this country and throughout the world. The need for specific groups for children, adolescents, women, and people of different socio-economic and ethnic backgrounds is becoming very important. Sensitivity to the population-specific issues of AIDS prevention, diagnosis, illness reactions, and grief must be reflected in how groups are planned and implemented (Getzel, 1991a; Child and Getzel, 1989). There can be no greater challenge. Although grief may weigh us down, the need for groups grows. Let us seek ways to face the demands ahead.

REFERENCES

Altman, L. K. (1991). WHO says 40 million will be infected with HIV by 2000. *The New York Times,* June 18, C, p. 3.

Camus, A. (1952). *The plague.* New York: Knopf.

Child, R. and Getzel, G. S. (1989). Group work with inner city people with AIDS. *Social Work with Groups*, 12(4), 65-80.

Children AIDS cases are reported to rise. (1990) *The New York Times,* September 26, A, p. 7.

Christ, G., Weiner, L., and Moynihan, R. (1986). Psychosocial issues in AIDS. *Psychiatric Annals,* 16, 173-179.

Erikson, E. H. (1964). *Insight and responsibility.* New York: W. W. Norton and Company.

Gambe, R. and Getzel, G. S. (1989). Group work with gay men with AIDS. *Social Casework,* 70(3), 172-179.

Getzel, G. S. (1991a). AIDS. In A. Gitterman (Ed.), *Handbook of social work with vulnerable populations* (pp. 35-64). New York: Columbia University Press.

Getzel, G. S. (1991b). Survival modes of people with AIDS in groups. *Social Work,* 36(1), 7-11.

Getzel, G. S. and Masters R. (1984). Serving families who survive homicide victims. *Social Casework,* 65, 138-144.

Getzel, G. S. and Mahony, K. (1990). Confronting human finitude: Group work with people with AIDS. *Journal of Gay and Lesbian Psychotherapy,* 1(3), 105-120.

Kramer, L. (1989). *Reports from the Holocaust.* New York: St. Martin's Press.

Lopez, D. J. and Getzel, G. S. (1984). Helping gay patients in crisis. *Social Casework,* 65, 387-394.

Lopez, D. J. and Getzel, G. S. (1986). Strategies for volunteers caring for persons with AIDS. *Social Casework,* 68, 47-53.

Navarro, M. (1990). AIDS foster care: Love and hope conquer fear. *The New York Times,* December 7, A, pp. 1,5.

Rounds, K. A., Galinsky, M. J., and Stevens L. S. (1991). Linking people with AIDS in rural communities: The telephone group. *Social Work,* 36(1), 13-18.

Shilts, R. (1988). *The band played on: Politics, people and AIDS.* New York: St. Martin's Press.

Yalom, I. (1984). *The theory and practice of group psychotherapy.* New York: Basic Books.

Chapter 4

Positive Group Work Experiences with African-American Adolescents 1935-1945: An Afrocentric Retrospective Analysis

Marjorie Witt Johnson

This chapter describes my experiences organizing and facilitating a modern dance group comprised of young, urban African-American adolescent girls between 1935 and 1945. More important, this chapter describes how I used social group work processes, methods, knowledge, African-American cultural norms, and modern dance to enhance the cultural identity, self-worth, and sense of confidence among a group of adolescent girls.

The conceptual framework for this chapter is the Afrocentric perspective. This perspective can best be defined as the process of analyzing and understanding African/African-American behaviors, attitudes, perceptions, values, and experiences from the cultural and historical vantage point of African/African-American people (Asante, 1990). The Afrocentric perspective also draws upon African culture and the unique historical experiences of African people throughout the diaspora for strategies and interventions to illuminate the myriad of social problems that plague African-American people (Asante, 1990).

I wish to acknowledge the support and assistance of the following people who were instrumental in the development of this paper: Paula Atwood, MSSA, LISW; Anthony E. O. King, PhD; Ruby Pernell, PhD; and Margaret Barry, MSW. I would also like to thank the Playhouse Settlement/Karamu Dancers who are living examples of the power of modern dance and social group work.

The Afrocentric perspective is the appropriate paradigm for this chapter because the motivation for the development of the Playhouse/Karamu dancers* came from my struggle to develop a positive cultural identity as a dark-skinned African-American girl and young adult.

Thus, my personal experiences, as well as the experiences of African-Americans in this country during the early 1920s and 1930s, had a tremendous impact upon my decision to participate in modern dance and to use it as an activity for enhancing positive group experiences for adolescent African-American girls.

Fifty-five years ago I did not know much, if anything, about African culture. Moreover, I did not know very much about the relationship between "Negro folk culture" and African culture. Today, with a greater awareness and knowledge of my African heritage and culture, I can reflect upon my work with the Playhouse/Karamu dancers and see that I was practicing social group work from an Afrocentric perspective. In addition, I now understand that many of the values and attitudes that formed the ethos for the Playhouse/Karamu dancers were essentially and fundamentally traditional African values.

From the benefit of hindsight, I now believe that the adolescent girls who participated in the Playhouse/Karamu dancers were attracted to modern dance because dance is and has always been an important activity in the spiritual and everyday lives of African/African-American people. In addition, our group experience was heavily influenced by several core African/African-American ideals: (1) the importance of the group; (2) the value of collective effort and cooperation; and (3) the importance of being genuine, open, and expressive in one's dealings with life (Nobles, 1985).

This chapter is an attempt to articulate the relationship between my work with adolescent African-American girls between 1935 and 1945 and the lessons I learned that can be applied in contemporary group work with urban African-American children and adolescents. This chapter is divided into five sections: (1) self-concept/skin color; (2) early, dance-group experiences; (3) processes such as

---

*The Playhouse Settlement dancers were renamed the Karamu dancers in 1939 after the Settlement House building was destroyed by fire. The word *Karamu* means "a place of joyful gathering" in KiSwahili.

decision making and personal interaction; (4) termination of the group; and (5) recommendations.

SELF-CONCEPT/ SKIN COLOR

My earliest recollection of my cultural/racial identity was that of being the darkest girl in a family of six. As a member of an African-American community in Cheyenne, a small town in Wyoming, I became aware of certain fundamental attitudes and beliefs regarding skin color. The darker a person's skin, the less attractive she or he was. Moreover, darker-skinned persons were perceived as being less intelligent and less capable than lighter-skinned persons. These attitudes and beliefs were formulated in the larger European-American society, but many African-Americans grew to accept them.

Although my self-concept was tainted by this badge of unattractiveness, my family provided me with enormous love, guidance, and support to help me cope. As a matter of fact, small groups of individuals and the general African-American community in which I grew up were active in supporting activities that contributed to my social, educational, and personal development. This assistance helped me cope with the negative attitudes associated with dark skin. As a consequence, I was able to avoid engaging in many self-defeating behaviors, such as skipping school and fighting because I might have been called racist names or been rejected by my peers. At the same time I was motivated to search for a positive sense of my cultural identity.

In college, although more exposed to racism than at any other time in my life, I found modern dance. Dancing helped me to deal with my badge of color because I learned how to use my total self in a positive way. I also developed a sense of confidence that influenced my attitudes toward other activities, particularly my academic work. When dancing I experienced freedom through running, leaping, falling, and recovering. I learned how to use my dark brown body in a unique, exhilarating way.

I had the opportunity to create dances that expressed the feelings surrounding my cultural/racial identity. Thus, I was given many opportunities to express my feelings and emotions in a special but important way. This entire experience taught me how modern dance or creative activities, in general, could be used to help an individual develop a positive cultural/racial identity and a level of self-confidence sufficient to influence one's achievements in other areas of life.

EARLY DANCE GROUP EXPERIENCES

The Playhouse Settlement in Cleveland, Ohio, offered a cultural arts education program that included activities such as drama, dance, and the visual arts. These activities were offered as tools for learning and developing social relationships within the neighborhood and the larger community. They also were centered around the talent and cultural traditions of African-Americans, which were called "Negro folk life," during that era. After graduating from college in 1935, I became a camp counselor for the Playhouse Settlement's summer camp.

The campers I supervised were 12 through 15 years of age. This camp provided children with two weeks in the open country and a variety of nature classes and cultural activities. The first meeting in the recreation hall started with six "finger snappin', feet tapping," enthusiastic African-American girls. These girls were acquainted with one another because they lived in the same neighborhoods. They had mastered the popular dance steps from their neighborhood, so I began by learning their dance routines.

During the evenings I had time to learn about their struggles to become accepted in their schools and neighborhoods. I also learned that they were experiencing some of the same problems associated with skin color and cultural identity that I had encountered. They were hurt when people called them "nappy headed" or "black so and so." They were also frustrated over being poor. All of these circumstances and burdens contributed to their dislike of school.

Although they were experiencing some of the same problems I had encountered growing up, they appeared to be more capable of coping with this problem because they were together as a group in their neighborhood. I shared my early struggles with them and what I had learned to do with my "total self" through modern dance. As we talked, practiced various dancing techniques, and engaged in creative improvisation to the sounds of well-known "Negro" spirituals, we began to bond. The girls performed during campfires for camp staff and other campers. Their performances were well received by the rest of the camp. The girls enjoyed modern dance and expressed a desire to continue when they returned to the Settlement. In my later research, I discovered that non-verbal activities are especially appropriate for adolescents (Middleman, 1968, 1990).

The first few years after camp, the six girls and I had problems becoming a part of the ongoing agency programs and finding space to continue the group. We solved these problems by deciding to meet in a nearby American Legion hall. Looking back, I now realize the "Negro" spirituals we danced, and the joy we experienced as we used improvisation to express our deeply and communally held beliefs and feelings fed our African/African-American consciousness.

I also realized that the motivation and need among young African-American adolescents to develop a positive sense of self as an African-American is strong. Moreover, I now realize that modern dance and other performing arts are an excellent medium for achieving a positive sense of self. Modern dance emphasizes the *group* experience and *social* relationships, two aspects of life that are culturally consistent with general African/African-American culture. Another aspect of our experience that was compatible with our cultural orientation was the level of spirituality we infused into our dancing. This spirituality, and our desire to express it in our creative dancing, was and is a major cultural norm among African/African-American people.

PROCESSES: DECISION MAKING AND PERSONAL INTERACTION

The first year after camp, the dancers and I began to develop a program of dances and activities in preparation for a presentation at their high school. Once the group was given permission and presented their dances at the school, they became known as the Playhouse Settlement Dance Group and were embraced as an important group within the agency. The performance at the high school also attracted new members for the dance group. Most important, their performance elicited the support of teachers at their high school, especially the history teachers. The history teachers demonstrated a renewed interest in the girls because their dances reflected the history of African-Americans, which was a point of interest for many instructors.

In essence, the teachers began to recognize some of the academic benefits modern dance experience produces. The group experience helped strengthen the girls' listening, thinking, problem solving, and decision-making skills. Creative movement and dance also helped them develop self-discipline, a quality required to perform well in the classroom.

At the same time the group was beginning to attract positive attention, I became a graduate social work student at the School of Applied Social Sciences (SASS) at (now Case) Western Reserve University. This is when I began to systematically unite creative dance with social group work. At SASS, I learned the importance of the group worker's role. Gertrude Wilson, one of my supervisors and instructors at SASS, stated that " . . . the quality of the group experience is dependent upon the skill of the worker to help members have a creative group experience as well as to acquire skills in various areas of program content" (Wilson and Ryland, 1949:179).

As our group flourished, I began to focus more attention on soliciting the support of the girls' families and communities. I spent many hours convincing the girls' family members of the social, academic, and psychological benefits of participating in modern dance activities. I also stressed the importance of family participation by encouraging family members to attend the group's performances.

The continued development of the now recognized Playhouse Settlement Dance Group demanded more planning and organizing than the girls and I had anticipated. We needed to deal with problems in the group-as-a-whole. Wilson and Ryland (1949) described this process as follows:

> Discussion and decision-making are vital to the composition of a dance. Each member may have ideas and while he or she may have to give up a "pet idea," the final content and form of the dance represent the integration of the ideas of many people–the goal of the whole group. The individual through this planning process and in the performance of the dance, feels the strength that comes from the group-as-a-whole. (p. 258-259)

Verbal exchanges with the members, listening to conversation and responses about techniques, improvisation, and performances, provided me with insight as to my role. Consequently, dance sessions were structured so that time was spent: (1) demonstrating techniques, (2) discussing and determining program themes or ideas, (3) developing program sequences, (4) rehearsing and perfecting techniques, (5) "spotting" individual members' difficulties and providing assistance (from the worker or another member), and (6) performing and assessing the quality of our performances. In subsequent readings and research, I discovered the structured approach was most helpful as the girls danced together in the group (Middleman, and Goldberg, 1974).

These dance sessions consisted of a great deal of interpersonal interaction, which enriched the members. Some members struggled for acceptance and status within the group as a whole. Grace Coyle (1940) discusses this concept of the interpersonal relationship as follows:

> The group leader, as he works with a group is aware not only of individuals as they participate in the multiform aspect of group life. He will also become aware of certain discernible processes by which individuals are related to each other. . . . Perhaps the most obvious to the observant leaders are the affectional relationships established between members of the group. (p. 71)

The manner in which we improvised the spiritual, "I'm a Rollin' through an Unfriendly World," is an example of the dynamics of interpersonal interaction in modern dance. The spiritual provided an opportunity for one member, moved by the story's idea in the song, to improvise on her feelings through a creative movement. Then other members would give their approval, by either commenting, or adding other movements to express their view of the story. As their group leader, I pulled these fragmented movements into a coherent dance routine that included everyone.

Creative movement as an idea became a motivating force for these dancers and for relationship building. The theme of the dance was used to guide the patterns of interaction. It was how members gained status and acquired different roles in the group-as-a-whole.

When the members reached consensus pertaining to a specific idea, there was generally a spirit of cooperation. Members were encouraged to be a part of the whole rather than having small cliques or sub-groups of individuals. The skilled or expressive dancers were encouraged to assist and guide others and build supportive relationships by working on dance ideas. By assisting others they increased their individual sense of value to the group. Since each member's creative involvement was based on ability and interest in being together, the collective results were perceived positively by everyone, including audiences.

The girls' unquestioning acceptance of these norms and expectations can be attributed to their traditional African-American culture, which emphasizes collective effort, mutual support and the importance of all individuals to the success of the group. One of the Karamu dancers (in 1939 the name of the group was changed from Playhouse Settlement Dancers), who is now involved in television in Los Angeles wrote the following in 1980:

> Through personal contact with each of us as members, and with all of the members in the group, we exchanged ideas and became like a family. Modern dance enriched our minds, broadened our mental outlook, and established self-confidence. We sweated, we worked, and stretched our imagination to the limit. To me, to perform was one of the greatest things I could do, because I loved it. I must have, I'm still doing it. (Interview with Royce Wallace)

The presentations and performances in the community were numerous over a three-year period. The group was in demand because they had become more than just a dance group. W. Gates, a writer for *Crossroad Magazine*, wrote in 1940 that the group had become "cultural historians."

> While working with the principles of modern dance the group is replenishing its African-American theme. Examining history pre and during slavery through the use of the spirituals has given this group the role of historians; their emotions, struggles, resentment and fight for freedom pervades the spirituals. Creative movement illuminates the song, and the song

enlarges the impact of the movement. . . . I cannot bid farewell to these dancers without making one more point; although they worked into the rehearsal a black wall, they seemed to dissolve it and move beyond a sea of faces, as though inspired from something within. The group has what I call a unique sense of communication. (W. Gates, p. 120)

The communication in the dance group was not based solely upon the members' common attachment to what they experienced together as historians. Because of their bonding, the dancers developed an esprit de corps that would last for decades (Coyle, 1979). Individual leaders emerged among the group based upon a wide range of abilities. Some dancers led because they possessed the ability to create new dance steps. Other dancers were able to assume leadership roles because they were superior technicians. Finally, other dancers were able to lead because they had the ability to reach within themselves and bring out the unique emotional quality of a dance that drew the group together as one and produced a powerful synergistic effect.

TERMINATION OF THE GROUP

The group, now called the Karamu Dancers, performed for many organizations and agencies. Their use of African-American culture as a basis for developing modern dance routines and programs had indeed made them historians, and they were in demand at universities, public schools, and "Negro" expositions in Pittsburgh and Detroit. One of the earliest highlights was when we appeared at the 1939 New York World's Fair.

After six years of performing, the needs of the agency and the group began to change, and, in some cases, conflict. For example, the agency's purposes and mission had become centered around fund raising for a new facility (the old building had burned down in 1939). Increased demands were made on the group to give benefit performances. At the same time, the members' needs had changed. Many began to search for employment and desired monetary compensation for their performances. Others wanted to further their education and dance training. Some actually left the group to attend college. The termination of the group was approaching.

The ending of this phase of the Karamu dancers required a long period of adjustment because of the depth of the relationships we had developed and the personal growth we had enjoyed. Brandler (1991) described the difficulties inherent in the termination process:

> The more profound the group experience, the more significant and meaningful the loss and the greater need for adjustment. In the ending phase, the importance of striking the right balance between preserving what has been gained by the group experience and successfully breaking away from the past can be underestimated. (p. 76-77)

As a worker, my mixed feelings were recognized and faced. There were numerous discussions about high points of success and areas of conflict and difficulties. Most important for some members was finding employment opportunities in dance companies and in shows on Broadway. Others found avenues for further education in college, while the remainder stayed with the agency and joined new members to continue the Karamu Dancers. Nevertheless, the original Playhouse Settlement Dancers had started a group that had by any standard achieved immense success. More important, they had pulled together, drawn by the lure of modern dance and a need to develop a healthy cultural identity, and enjoyed a positive growth-enhancing experience that would stay with them for the rest of their lives.

RECOMMENDATIONS

This chapter has dealt primarily with the African-American adolescent and the importance of knowing the trials and tribulations of their ancestors, particularly the efforts they made to overcome the obstacles they encountered. If they do not know who they are and their history, then they can become alienated from their roots and the knowledge acquired over many generations and hundreds of years (King, 1991).

I feel that all youth could benefit from participating in the discipline of modern dance, which is a kinesthetic modality. Therefore, I recommend that children in grades 4 through 12 have an opportunity to experience modern dance and enjoy the benefits it can provide. I also feel that school social workers and public school teachers should consider using modern dance as a school-based intervention. Graduate schools of social work and education should offer courses that provide the knowledge and skills required to use this model to enhance growth options and resolve social and academic problems. In addition, social science researchers need to study the effects of this approach on the psychosocial growth and development of children and adolescents. We need to identify the types of experiences and the conditions and circumstances in which this model produces the desired outcomes.

Social workers who are skilled group workers and community organizers should be at the forefront of this important movement. They would understand and appreciate the benefits of the group experience. In addition, social workers are trained to locate and coordinate resources and link systems that appear on the surface to have no relationship to one another. Most of these tasks require vision, creativity, knowledge of the community, and a commitment to the well-being of children and their families. Who possesses more of these qualities than social workers?

REFERENCES

Asante, M. K. (1990). *Afrocentricity.* Trenton, NJ: Africa World Press, Inc.

Brandler, S. (1991). *Group skills and strategies for effective interventions.* New York: The Haworth Press, Inc.

Coyle, G. L. (1940). *Group work with American youth.* New York: Harper & Row.

Coyle, G. L. (1979). *Social processes and organized groups.* Hebron, CT: Practitioners Press, Inc.

Gates, W. (1940). Of the People: A Negro Group Turns to Folk Song for Emotional Stuff of the Dance. *Crossroad Magazine,* (Cleveland, Spring 1940), p. 120.

Johnson, M. Witt. (1943). Social group worker with adolescents at Playhouse Settlement. Unpublished thesis, advised by Grace L. Coyle, Professor of Group Work at Case Western Reserve School of Applied Social Sciences (now Mandel School of Applied Social Science).

King, A. E. O. (1992). Racial consciousness and social behavior; a response to the impact of black consciousness on health and social behavior of African-American males. In L. E. Gary and M. V. Mbanaso (Eds.). *Proceedings of the Conference on Health and Social Behavior of African-American Males,* pp. 341-348. Washington, DC Institute of Urban Affairs and Research, Howard University.

Middleman, R. (1968). *The non-verbal method of working with groups*. New York: Associated Press.

Middleman, R (1990). Group work and the Heimlich Maneuver: Unchoking social work education. *Plenary Address, 12th Symposium, Association for the Advancement of Social Work with Groups, Miami, FL, October 28, 1990.*

Middleman, R. and Goldberg, G (1974). *Social service delivery: A structural approach to social work practice*. NY: Columbia University Press.

Nobles, W. W. (1985). Black Family Life: A Theoretical and Policy Implication Literature Review. In A. R. Harvery (Ed.). *The black family: Afrocentric perspective*. NY: United Church Commission for Racial Justice.

Wallace, R. (1980). Personal conversation with author.

Wilson, G. and Ryland, G. (1949). *Social group work practice*. Cambridge, MA: University Press.

Chapter 5

The New Patient Mix:
Group Work and Chronic Disorders
in an Acute Care Hospital

Patricia Moffat
Noreen Kay

THE SETTING

Sunnybrook Health Science Centre is a University of Toronto teaching hospital, situated in a large metropolitan area. It has 600 acute care beds providing a full range of services to adults. Emergency and outpatient service is provided with specialized units for trauma, HIV/AIDS, nephrology, and cardiovascular surgery, as well as a regional cancer center. The population in the hospital's catchment area is stable and suburban and includes many frail elderly people living in their own homes. Originally a veterans hospital, Sunnybrook also has 600 beds on the same site providing long-term care to entitled veterans.

The Department of Social Work has 45 workers organized into five teams: four in acute care–surgery, medicine, psychiatry, oncology–and one Extended Care team for veterans long-term care. In 1991, an inventory of current, inactive, and planned group work programs in the department was compiled to facilitate staff training, program development, and student field instruction. This chapter will analyze the new patient mix and illustrate the differential use of group work in an acute care setting.

THE NEW PATIENT MIX

In the 1990s, chronic disorders are a feature of acute care hospital programs. The population is aging, and patients have serial hospital admissions and treatment events, but they and their families require medical supervision and social support over a long period of time. Many clients are community-living adults with diabetes, cancer, heart disease, or kidney failure. In some cases, this is compounded by the slow physical and cognitive decline of Parkinson's, Alzheimer's, multi-infarct dementia, and other progressive disorders. Social isolation of the frail elderly and lack of adequate community support services are major problems confronting Sunnybrook social workers in providing service to the new patient mix. In many situations, group work is not an add-on to regular social work services, it is the intervention of choice

RELATIVE GROWTH OF THREE
GROUPS OF ELDERLY

The profile of the population over age 65 is changing rapidly. A 1990 Ontario provincial report estimated the growth of three groups of elderly between 1983 and 2011. The group age of 65 to 74 will increase 78.9 percent, the 75 to 84 group will increase 122.9 percent, and the people age 85 and older will increase in numbers 222.0 percent. (Elderly Services Branch, Ministry of Community and Social Services).

Canada has 9 percent of elderly in institutions, compared with 4 or 5 percent in the United Kingdom and the United States. With the rapid growth of the 85-plus age group, length of stay in long-term care is increasing, so beds are not available for the two younger groups of elderly until their care needs are very heavy. This places a heavier burden on home support services and family caregivers. The youngest group of elderly have increasing responsibility for their 85-plus elderly parents. This is a new and highly vulnerable group of caregivers, when contrasted with the popular image of the caregiving adult child as an active, employed, middle-aged person of the female persuasion.

There are also signs of a new generation gap, a conflict of values between the younger and older groups of elderly. Yet, all the elderly share a need to maintain control over decision making, hence, the increased interest in living wills and advance health care directives (Molloy and Guyatt, 1991). As people grow older, they fear slipping into the "post-adult" status where others, often professionals, make decisions on their behalf (Matthews, 1979).

WHO IS HELPING COMMUNITY RESIDENTS 55 AND OLDER?

In its 1985 general survey, Statistics Canada inquired about the provision of in-home assistance to community residents aged 55 and older (Table 5.1).

TABLE 5.1. Distribution of Sources of Assistance with Activities of Daily Living for Community Residents Aged 55 and Over

Total formal organization sources	7.4%
Total Informal Sources	92.6%
Spouse	49.83%
Daughter	23.4%
Son	7.4%
Other Relative	4.41%
Friend/neighbor	4.58%

Statistics Canada, General Social Survey, 1985.

Only 7.4 percent of help with activities of daily living is provided by formal organizations, and almost 50 percent is given by spouses. An increasing number of these spouse caregivers are themselves elderly, frail, and in poor health. A recent American Association of Retired Persons (AARP) survey (1987) estimated "the average length of home care for a severely dependent person over 70 is between 5 and 6 years. In many cases the caregivers are only slightly more able than the dependents." Elder care is a major source of stress in family life, and its long-term emotional and economic demands increase the risk of neglect or even abuse of the elderly.

SOCIAL AND LIFESTYLE FACTORS
IN ELDER CARE

In addition to their *longer lives* and the increased incidence of *chronic disease*, our present patient mix has a *lower ratio of children to parents*. In 1900, there were 13.6 adults between 18 and 64 for every person over 65. In 1990, the ratio was 4.8 to 1.

In terms of the work force, we are also seeing a lower support ratio for the elderly. If you retired in 1935, 40 workers contributed to your pension; in 1950, 17 workers; and in 1990, 3.4 workers. In 2020, when the postwar children retire, only 1.78 workers will contribute to the pension of each retiree (Dychtwald and Flower, 1989).

The greater lifespan of women has lead to a great increase in widowhood. Because men tend to remarry younger women, elderly poverty and social isolation has a predominantly female face (Cohen, 1984).

The *increased entry of women* of caregiving age *into the labor force* not only erodes the supply of unpaid family caregivers, it also adds a third job to women already handling full time employment, homemaking, and child care. Elder care is appearing only recently as an item in workplace benefit packages and union contract demands (Work and Family Survey, CARNET, 1993).

SOCIAL GROUP WORK IN HEALTH CARE

Social work intervention in health care occurs at a point of crisis and/or transition when the client and their family realize that there is no going back to "the way things were" in the past. To the clients, the social worker has a commitment to review their options for care and their coping style, to strive for an acceptable balance in the sharing of family responsibility for physical, social, and financial care. Patients need to be involved in decisions that affect their future. Viewing the clients in their social matrix, the worker knows that this process can stir up old conflicts among family members, but it can also bring them closer together. Models like Edith Moore's "kith and kin" approach help us to have a vision of the client's social environment beyond the simple listing of blood relatives (Moore, 1991).

The need for advocacy is never clearer than in situations where clients lack legally sanctioned relationships by blood or marriage. Clients can also be marginalized by immigrant or refugee status, poverty, or the simple lack of effort by the system to overcome the language and cultural barriers to effective care and client autonomy in decision making.

In the multi-disciplinary team, the social worker's role is as a mediator and "trouble-shooter" for clients perceived as different, non-compliant, or otherwise problematic. She or he is also mandated to ensure continuity of care. This involves client and agency liaison within the hospital and the community, knowledge of resources for ongoing care, and support after discharge. Less prominent, but equally important is follow-up study and research to evaluate the effectiveness of these interventions and ensure that future programs take account of the social and cultural features of our new patient mix.

Social workers acknowledge the strength and leadership that come from members of a group. The programs we will present all encourage and facilitate leadership and problem solving by members as the group goes through its stages of development (Garland, Jones, and Kolodny, 1976). In health care, leadership is often shared, and the social worker must engage a parallel group, the multi-disciplinary team, in supporting and participating in the group's contribution to recovery and continuing care. Workers must also maintain for colleagues the vision of the patient in their social matrix, so that "admissions" and "treatment events" are seen in the context of long-term health care and social support for people with chronic disorders. They are conscious always of the organizational barriers to continuity of care in a setting designed to deliver a "high-tech," episode style of service.

THREE GROUP WORK APPROACHES
IN ACUTE CARE

In our description of three group work approaches to the new patient mix in acute care, we will show how group work concepts can be adapted to this setting and population. In the Sunnybrook Diabetes Education Centre (SUNDEC) program, medical imperatives and information are presented to patients diagnosed with diabetes. In the cardiac spouse's group, the vision of the patient in their social matrix is shared with family members and with staff on the surgical service to enhance follow-up and continuing care. The third program, a support group for oncology staff, enhances competency and team support in a service for cancer patients in acute and terminal stages of the disease.

A HEALTH EDUCATION GROUP
FOR DIABETICS

The SUNDEC program is designed to provide support and education to diabetic patients and their families. The program takes the form of a two-day workshop in which members of the health care team present information to the group on a variety of topics as, for example, what is diabetes, diet, exercise, stress management, and living with diabetes. The staff uses a mixed format of films, lectures, and discussion in the group. Referrals come from many sources including the family physician, diet specialists, information in the media, and self-referrals.

The group is facilitated by a social worker who acts as a moderator. The group members are asked to introduce themselves and identify concerns they have about living with diabetes or living with someone who is diabetic. The workshop takes place in what can be described as a "user-friendly" setting. The meeting room resembles a reception area or living room. Participants sit in a circle rather than in rows. These factors combined with the informal style of the staff promote an environment that is conducive to discussion and sharing.

The use of the group work method works well because participants are able to see that chronic illness is a family issue. There is a delicate interplay between how the patient deals with the illness and how those close to them deal with it. However, the message that is reinforced is that although family support is important, the primary responsibility for managing the diabetes falls on the patient. People with chronic illness, especially newly diagnosed patients, often have a sense that they are abnormal. Coming together as a group gives them an opportunity to normalize themselves and their experience. It allows them not to become isolated in their illness.

Living with diabetes poses challenges related to lifestyle and dietary changes and the need to take medication and monitor blood sugars. Group members often complain that they are restricted from engaging in pleasurable activities, such as going out to dinner or taking a vacation. In the program, they learn that they can still do these things and comply with the requirements of managing their diabetes. They learn from each other's creative ways of living with their illness. They have support to face the challenges of diabetes from others who understand their experience of chronic illness because they too are living it. This process empowers the group members to reclaim the control they feel they have lost in their lives and it instills hope and understanding that the quality of their life will be altered but not destroyed by chronic illness.

A significant feature of the SUNDEC program is the follow-up sessions that group members are invited to attend. These half-day sessions take place approximately three to four months after the initial seminar and are open-ended. Attendance is voluntary and patients and families can attend as often as they like. The follow-up sessions provide an opportunity for participants to touch base again and encourages them to keep motivated. The material discussed serves as a kind of refresher course for the original workshop, and members can learn of new advances in the area of their disease. Most of the population this group serves is middle-aged or older. Patients report a benefit from hearing the information repeated, as it allows them to connect and integrate it more effectively. For many elderly patients living alone, attendance at the follow-up sessions has a social purpose.

Perhaps the success of this group can be best summed up in this excerpt from a letter that was sent to hospital administration about the SUNDEC program:

I was having trouble coming to terms with the fact I had been diagnosed as having the dreaded disease called *diabetes* and that a lifestyle change was necessary to control it. When I arrived Monday morning, I was deeply depressed and upset with myself and my diagnosis. But, the comprehensive two-day seminar answered all my questions, helped me come to terms with the fact that I had diabetes, made me feel positive about myself, and left me with the feeling that I can control it versus it controlling me. I learned diet control, better eating habits, the benefit of exercise, how to test my blood, etc., but most of all I learned that I am not alone in this and that I have a support system to help me deal with diabetes. I want to stress how important this program was to me (and will be in the future as it continues to give me the guidance and support I need–plus the guilt complex I need to make me lose weight) and how, in these recessionary times, this is definitely not an area that should be cut back or cut out. I am sure I can speak for others when I say that by offering this support for us, you are helping to keep us from getting out of control and becoming a burden on the health care system.

CARDIAC SPOUSES: A SUPPORT GROUP WITH STAFF EDUCATION FEATURES

On the cardiovascular surgery service, a support and education group for spouses or partners of discharged cardiovascular patients has become an integral part of the program. The spouses are the focus of our group work because the literature suggests that the spouse's reaction to the cardiac event influences the patient's recovery as it relates to regimen compliance and life adjustment (Miller and Wikoff, 1989).

The group takes place approximately three to six months following the patient's surgery. The rationale for this timing is that three to six months represents a transitional stage in the patient's recovery as the initial crisis and post-operative phase is over and patients are usually able to return to work and/or begin to resume other activities.

The groups run for six weekly sessions of one and a half hours, and group membership is closed by the second meeting. The group is led by a female social worker and the female clinical nurse specialist (CNS) on the cardiovascular service. This provides a good balance as the CNS takes responsibility for imparting medical information, but is also very empathic and holistic in her approach to the individual.

The group is based on a reciprocal model of social group work using a humanistic perspective (Alissi, 1980). The role of the group leaders is to facilitate discussion and this is achieved through a variety of means—written material, presentations, use of videos, inviting guest speakers, homework exercises, and experiential role play.

A significant feature of this group is a questionnaire that is mailed to potential group members prior to the group's first meeting. The questionnaire identifies areas in their lives in which they might be experiencing difficulty. It serves several purposes for the group leaders. It gives us greater insight into areas of concern that individuals might not feel comfortable discussing in a group, it helps identify themes, and it can be used as a baseline means of comparison for research purposes. For the group members, the questionnaire helps to process some of the potential issues of the group ahead of time, so they have specific reasons for wanting to join.

Some of the issues identified in questionnaires included concerns around compliance with rehabilitation programs, problems in the relationship, concerns about future cardiac problems, fear of losing their partner emotionally or physically, fear of being alone, sadness over limits to social or recreational activity, and having to take on new roles and responsibilities at a time when the spouses are also aging. Many persons reported trying to "shield" their partner from information for fear of provoking a heart attack. Another common report was of needing someone "to explode to" without feeling disloyal.

Because of the limited number of sessions, it is necessary to help the group members move through the stages of the group process as quickly as possible. In the first meeting, participants are asked to introduce themselves and are encouraged to share their cardiac story and identify themselves as a cardiac spouse. Common themes are identified in the group, and the group members decide which topics they wish to work on in future sessions.

Group content is decided democratically by the membership and each series of meetings has had a somewhat different focus. For example, one group was heavily focused on emotional reactions after the surgery. We found that spouses' reactions often mirrored those of the patients. We looked at anger, depression, and fear extensively.

Another group was interested in exploring areas of stress and its management. My most recent group examined personality changes after surgery and improved methods of communication.

All groups chose to spend part or all of one session addressing medical questions. The nutritionist was asked to present to three of the groups and, on two occasions, organized a shopping tour at a nearby supermarket in which she explained package labels and answered questions about food selection and dietary habits.

The system of mutual aid that developed in most groups was noteworthy. There was almost a family-like relationship in several of the groups and a sense of respect as group members learned from each other (Lang, 1991). The age of the participants varied, and often older group members could share their life experience and coping strategies with younger members to great effect. The system of mutual aid was also apparent in expressions of concern at a group member's absence, the tendency of several group members to remain behind and continue talking with each other after sessions, and the exchange of telephone numbers that took place at termination of several of the groups (Gitterman and Shulman, 1986).

For the participants, their experience of living with a partner with heart disease was normalized and their feelings about it validated. Group members recognized that they were in a safe environment to share their concerns. This was empowering for them and inspired a sense of hopefulness that there would still be quality to their lives and that they were not alone.

As the group meetings took place in a conference room on the cardiovascular service, the nurses became very curious about what was taking place in our meetings. Consequently, last spring the two group leaders gave a series of presentations to the nursing staff and multi-disciplinary team about the groups and the kinds of issues that were being identified as stressful for the spouses. Confidentiality of group members was strictly respected.

The presentations provided an additional benefit from the use of group work in that they helped the multi-disciplinary team to have a vision of the patient in their social matrix. So much attention is focused on the patient during the brief stay in hospital. Those close to the patient, most notably the spouse or partner, are often in the shadows. The presentations helped the team understand the patients in the context of their other relationships and how these relationships can influence their regimen, compliance, and life adjustment to promote a more positive outcome and recovery.

ENHANCING COMPETENCY AND MUTUAL SUPPORT: A STAFF GROUP IN ONCOLOGY

An interesting example of the use of group work concepts and methods in acute care takes place on the oncology service. Early in 1992, a multidisciplinary staff support group was formed at the suggestion of the team social worker. Its formation was based on the premise that, in order to be helpful to the patient, it is important to start with a healthy staff.

An identified problem with staff on the oncology service was high turnover, especially among nurses. Many of the nurses were young, often new graduates. Dealing with death and dying was difficult. The group leader described a case of a 22-year-old nurse who felt conflicted about helping people end their life at a time when hers was just beginning.

Groups had been tried on the oncology service in the past, but were unsuccessful. The idea of a support group was too threatening to staff, as there were fears of a lack of confidentiality and being viewed as unable to cope by their peers. What makes this group work well is that it is framed as a competency-enhancing vehicle. The description of its purpose states that it is "to facilitate positive inter-professional behavior, enhance oncology multi-disciplinary education, and encourage mutual support." The group provides a forum for sharing patient-related concerns, enhancing work relations and improving and maintaining morale.

All members of the multi-disciplinary team, including staff physicians, occupational therapy, physiotherapy, chaplaincy, pharmacy, and the home care coordinator were invited to attend. There is good representation from all disciplines. Meetings take place monthly at lunch time. The group is open-ended and is run by the social worker and the clinical nurse specialist, who act as organizers and facilitators. Group members are asked to sign a confidentiality contract before joining.

Each meeting has a theme and the format of the group is a lecture or presentation, followed by group discussion. Some of the group members have given presentations related to their discipline. At other times, guest speakers are brought in. Topics have included ethical issues: DNR (do not resuscitate) and hydration of the terminally ill, stress in the workplace, humor therapy, role of the occupational and physical therapist (OT/PT), and professional grief. Attendance is usually ten to fifteen people and the group may need to find a larger room for its meetings.

This oncology program is an innovative group that is still in the early stages of its development. The responses from evaluation forms to date have provided some useful feedback. Participants report finding the information presented very useful. They have learned new things and they have requested more information on specific topics. Other comments have related to a better understanding of team members' roles, a realization that "not only nurses have bad days" and reports of the benefits of getting to know other team members on a personal level.

CONCLUSIONS

The new patient mix in acute care presents a challenge to a hospital system designed primarily to provide emergency and episodic health care. The present and future patient population is aging and characterized by chronic and progressive disorders and disabilities. Social workers need to assess patients in their social matrix and work collaboratively with institutional and community colleagues to facilitate continuity of care. The active involvement of patients and families in planning and decision making is central to the worker's role in advocacy and community liaison. Changes in demography, economics, and family care resources were reviewed, along with our need to share a vision of the patient as part of a network of "kith and kin" within the patient's environment.

Social group work is often the intervention of choice with this population in an acute care setting. Group work involves a mixture of education and mutual support to assist in problem definition, coping with losses, life review, learning about resources, adapting to changing roles and tasks, and facing the future with a different lifestyle and social network.

Groupwork is a proactive approach that enhances team work, client autonomy, and continuity of care. Three programs in acute care were presented to illustrate the application of group work concepts and methods to the health care and social support needs of the new patient mix and their family and institutional caregivers.

Issues in multi-disciplinary team work, staff education, and shared leadership were also identified. The need for more follow-up care and program evaluation was emphasized, in order to establish a database for organizational and political change that will respond to the future health care needs of an aging population with chronic disorders and declining social and economic resources.

REFERENCES

AARP. *Domestic Mistreatment of the Elderly: Towards Prevention.* Washington, DC: Criminal Justice Services, 1987.

Cohen, Leah. *Small Expectations: Society's Betrayal of Older Women.* Toronto: McLelland and Stewart, 1984.

Dychtwald, K. and Flower, J. *Age Wave: The Challenges of an Aging North America.* Los Angeles: Jeremy Tarcher, Inc., 1989.

Garland, J., Jones, H., and Kolodny, R. A Model for Stages of Development in Group Work. S. Bernstein (Ed.). *Explorations in Group Work: Theory and Practice.* Boston: Charles River Books, 1976.

Gitterman, Alex and Shulman, Lawrence (Eds.). *Mutual Aid Groups and the Life Cycle.* IL: Peacock Publishers, 1986.

Lang, Norma. *The Family-like Group: A Powerful Entity in Social Work Practice with Groups.* AASWG 13th Symposium, Akron, Ohio, 1991.

Matthews, Sarah H. *The Social World of Old Women: Management of Self-Identity.* Sage Library of Social Research, 1979.

Miller, P. J. and Wikoff, R. Spouses' Psychosocial Problems, Resources and Marital Functioning Postmyocardial Infarction. *Progress in Cardiovascular Nursing,* 4 (April-June): 71-76, 1989.

Molloy, D. William and Guyatt, Gordon H. A Comprehensive health care directive in a home for the aged. *Canadian Medical Association Journal,* 145(4): xx-xx, 1991.

Moore, Edith E. *Vision and Voice in Kith and Kin Groups: Bringing Society Back Home.* 13th AASWG Symposium, Akron, Ohio, October, 1991.

Work & Family: The Survey. The Work & Eldercare Research Group: CARNET. Gulph, Ontario: The Canadian Aging Research Network, 1993.

Chapter 6

Bringing the Mountain to Mohammed: An Experiential Approach to Teaching Group Dynamics in the Classroom

Marcia B. Cohen

The trend away from specialization by method in social work education presents challenges to the teaching of social group work. Practice theory and skills are increasingly being taught across method areas within generalist curricula, posing the danger of group work content becoming diluted or lost. Where group experiences are not routinely available in field practice, this threat is intensified.

Faculty teaching group work course content must be innovative to ensure that students have "real-life" group experiences to which their theoretical learning can be applied. A review of the group work course syllabi available at AASWG's 1991 annual symposium suggests that student task groups are frequently used for this purpose. This teaching tool brings the small group experience into the classroom, providing a laboratory in which group dynamics can be experienced, observed, and analyzed. There has been, however, been little discussion of this experiential approach in the social work literature. What has been written focuses primarily on the use of task groups in research rather than practice courses (Latting and Raffoul, 1991).

This chapter will discuss a task group assignment used in a Master's level group work course. The assignment was designed to strengthen students' learning of group dynamics content, including roles, norms, interactional patterns, and group development (Toseland and Rivas, 1984; Garland, Jones, and Kolodny, 1976).

EDUCATIONAL SETTING AND COURSE ASSIGNMENT

"Social Work Practice with Groups" is part of the second-year practice curriculum in an MSW program. The program offers a generalist foundation curriculum and two second-year concentrations: Clinical Practice and Practice Management. The group practice course is required of all students and includes content on work with groups across the practice continuum from treatment groups to task groups. More than one-third of the students taking the course do not have a concurrent group assignment in their fieldwork. Some have had no prior group experience.

The course assignment consists of a task group project and an individual log. Students form small groups based on their interests in specific types of groups (activity groups, educational groups, etc.). Each student group is charged with the task of leading a class session on their particular group approach. The student groups meet throughout the semester to work on this task.

Students use their logs to record systematic observations of the emergence and interplay of group roles, norms, and interactional patterns during the course of group development. Completed logs include a comprehensive summary and assessment of group structure and development, applying literature on group processes to the task group experience.

During the 1992 spring semester, the author taught two sections of Social Work Practice with Groups to a total of 45 students. Each course section divided into four groups with the task of presenting a class session on one of four topics: therapy groups, activity groups, educational groups, and task groups.

The group formation process consisted of the instructor writing the four topics on the blackboard and asking students to identify the group they would like to join. Decisions were based, for the most part, on student interest in a particular group approach. Some students also considered who the other group members would be before making their decisions, attempting to join with friends, or avoid least favorite classmates.

Once the mechanics of group formation were completed, the groups began to meet. One hour of class time was available weekly for group meetings. The instructor was available on a consultative basis. Each group had seven (in some cases, eight) weeks to prepare their class presentation. During this period, members recorded their observations of the unfolding group processes in their logs.

The student logs provide vivid accounts of the group experience and reflect the learning potential in this assignment. Excerpts from the logs will be used below to illustrate student learning in four areas: roles, norms, interactional patterns, and group development. Although these will be presented as discrete processes for didactic purposes, the logs themselves reflect the complex interplay of these dynamics.

ROLES

Group roles have been defined as shared expectations about behavior patterns and the function of individuals in the group (Northen, 1988; Toseland and Rivas, 1984). These contextual roles (Radin and Feld, 1985) reflect a complex interplay between individual and group dynamics. Certain roles, such as leader, gatekeeper, compromiser, and scapegoat emerged in almost all the groups. The role of leader was commented on most often in the student logs.

Group 1 was plagued by leadership conflicts from its inception. With eight members, it was the largest group. These students joined the group out of a common interest in therapy groups, with little consideration of group composition. Joan was one group member who considered composition, although not decisively. In her first journal entry she states:

> I was strongly attracted to joining the group therapy task group as this is the direction I feel I need to go in and want more knowledge of. When I looked on the blackboard and noticed all the very strong egos in the group I thought about switching to another group. But, I finally decided to stay in this group. I did not think I would be one of the strong egos. . . .

Group 1 consisted of five women and three men, all between the ages of 30 and 45. As Joan's entry suggests, a number of these students were outspoken in class and were dominant members of the student community. As Joan anticipated, leadership conflicts were evident from the beginning:

> Less than 3 minutes after we began our first meeting, the leadership role was being vied for. Donald made a statement about the direction the group should go in and Juliana quickly asked him "are you the leader?" Donald withdrew after that and the leadership conflict shifted to Juliana and Greg, with each of them acting as though they were trying to get the rest of the group to accept them as the leader. I silently asked myself why I did not get out of this group when I had the chance.

Over the course of group development, the leadership role shifted several times. Most often it was shared between Ruth in the role of task leader and Rosie in the role of socio-emotional leader (Northen, 1988). Neither of these women engaged in the initial leadership struggles with Donald, Juliana, and Greg. Ruth was a bright, articulate woman in her forties, highly respected by her classmates. Rosie was a shy young woman who did not excel academically. Joan analyzes the roles that emerged in Group 1.

> Initially Donald, Greg, and Juliana actively vied for leadership. None of them were really accepted as leaders by the group, and Donald and Greg eventually withdrew, missing meetings and becoming uninvested in the group. They both became scapegoats for the group.
>
> When the content of group meetings became affective, Rosie was the socio-emotional leader. Usually very quiet, when she would get angry she would speak up. It was Rosie who forced the group to examine its own process and talk about feelings.
>
> Ruth functioned as the group's task leader. I often thought she assumed this role to diffuse the heavy, emotional conflicts and redirect our attention to the task at hand. Ruth was also in the role of gatekeeper, keeping the group moving forward and

away from deep, emotionally laden material. Surprisingly, there were no conflicts between Rosie and Ruth. The group really needed both of them.

Ruth examined her own role in the group in her log summary:

> Leadership was a multilevel issue in this group. I felt that I was the internal leader even though we rotated the role of group facilitator every week. I suggested the idea of rotating the facilitator and it became my role each week to suggest someone to be the facilitator. In this sense, I manifested the internal leadership role over and over.

Group 2 experienced fewer leadership conflicts than Group 1 had and generally had a more fluid role structure. The group was composed of six females and one male, ranging in age from mid-thirties to mid-forties. The group formation process for Group 2 was somewhat unique. Two groups of three students each had approached one another, prior to the class session in which task groups were formed, and decided to work together. Preferences for group topic were expressed, but were not particularly strong. In class, these six students volunteered to be in the task group focused on activities groups. They were joined by a seventh student, Iris. Group 2 was formed out of the mutual attraction of its members rather than the topic.

Serena, a Group 2 member in her 40s, described the roles she observed in the group:

> In regards to the indigenous leadership role, there were several members who tried to take that position during our early group meetings (Barb, Iris, Kara, and myself). Iris and Kara were frequently in the leadership role as the group developed but at times other members shared that role with them.
> When Kara became very negative about the group, she was cast in the role of deviant group member.
> At times Barb was the group scapegoat. Fay was the quiet member, always cooperative, but rarely initiating anything. Lori was in the role of encourager at times. She also served as the gatekeeper along with Iris. Jimmy played the role of compromiser during many of the group meetings. I wonder if he

gravitated to this role because he was the only male member in the group? Jimmy was also in the deviant role when he did not do his group homework assignment on time. I was most often in the role of procedural technician but at times I shared the leadership role with Kara and Iris.

Barb paints a vivid picture of emerging leadership in Group 2 as it was acted out during a walk to the library:

> The group decided to meet in the library. Kara said she knew a really nice room where we could meet. We walked to the library in single file, laughing and enjoying ourselves. Kara was our leader and we were pretending to be ducks. Jimmy was making duck noises and we were having great fun. We walked all the way to the library like that, in line behind Kara.

NORMS

Norms have been defined as shared expectations about the proper and acceptable ways to act in a group, reflecting value judgments about behavior (Northen, 1988; Toseland and Rivas, 1984). The most clearly identifiable norms in the student task groups revolved around such issues as what would and would not be discussed in the group, how absences from group meetings would be handled, how group members would be held accountable for their specific task assignments, and how group decisions would be made.

In many of the groups, examination of group process and direct expression of feelings were taboo. This was particularly evident in Group 3 whose focus was educational groups. This group was composed of six members, all women in their thirties. Despite their apparent homogeneity, group members saw themselves as embodying irreconcilable differences.

Beth, in her late thirties, observed her friend, Caroline, attempt to raise process issues in several group meetings:

> Caroline tried to talk about the group dynamics again in today's meeting but again her effort to get the group to ex-

amine its process failed. I tried to help but the norm against talking about what is happening is just too strong. Apparently one of our norms is not to discuss what our norms are! Myra and Sylvie, especially, enforce this norm. Each time Caroline tried to bring up what was happening in the group, Myra would interrupt or begin a side conversation with Sylvie.

Beth might have been surprised to see a similar observation in Myra's log:

> Yalom states that norms can be either explicit or implicit (1985). Our group had a number of implicit norms. One of the earliest norms was "never talk directly about the group process." A related norm was "do not explore your feelings within the group." We all participated in this conspiracy of silence, to the detriment of the group.

Group 5, also focused on educational groups, developed a very different norm. This group consisted of two women in their late twenties and two men in their mid-forties. All four were attracted to the group based on its topical focus. Group 5 evolved a norm of sharing feelings and reflections openly. Alyssa discussed this norm in her log summary:

> Daniel and Jim had been locked in a power struggle during our first two group meetings. Instead of letting this sabotage group process, Daniel risked talking about his feelings. Jim responded by talking about his feelings and about the anger he had experienced from Daniel. Daniel told Jim that he did not feel so angry anymore, now that they were talking about it.
>
> I thought it was fascinating that instead of there being an unspoken power struggle between the two men it was now out in the open and could be resolved. I told them it felt good that they could share their feelings, that it was good role modeling for the group.

Jimmy, the lone male member in Group 2, discovered the strength of a group norm when he violated it. Two weeks before the group presentation, Jimmy came unprepared to a group meeting:

One powerful norm was that of responsibility to the group, particularly in terms of following through on commitments. I discovered that I had violated this norm when I arrived to the sixth group meeting minimally prepared to rehearse my part of the presentation. Although there were no heavy consequences for this infringement, I felt the strong pressure of the group. I understood that there were certain expectations I had to meet as a member of the group in order for us to fulfill our group goals.

All of the groups evolved norms for decision making. For most groups, the explicit norm was one of decision making by consensus; however, the groups operationalized the concept of consensus decision making very differently. Group 6 agreed on decision through consensus in their first group meeting. The five women in this group, who ranged in age from 35 to 50, were deeply committed to feminism and egalitarian group functioning. Portia, the eldest group member, discussed what the norm of consensus meant for Group 6:

> When I use the word *consensus* I do not mean the kind of unanimity that comes when it is made difficult or impossible for someone to express a different opinion or reservation. I also do not mean that all differences are ignored. The way it worked in our group, consensus was the acceptance of what seemed to everyone to be the best decision in a given situation. It was arrived at only after a thorough attempt to explore all positions, alternatives, and feelings.

Consensus decision making in Group 2 was quite different, as Joan's description reveals:

> Decisions in the group came quickly, usually on the heels of someone pushing their idea hard and the group needing to decide something so that we could move forward. We always operated by consensus but at times it seemed like the kind of consensus that comes from bullying. . . . Often we embraced whatever idea was on the table, any idea at all. Many of the things we decided were never followed through on at all.

INTERACTIONAL PATTERNS

Helen Northen (1988) defines *social interaction* as " . . . the dynamic interplay of forces in which the contact between persons results in a modification of the behavior and attitudes of the participants" (p. 22). She views communication, both verbal and nonverbal, as " . . . the very essence of social interaction . . . " (p. 22). Students were generally able to identify their group's interactional style as fitting one or more of the patterns described in the literature. Group 4, focused on task groups and consisting of two women in their middle twenties and two women in their late forties, evolved an interactional pattern that worked well for this small group. Sydney, one of the older women in the group, provided the following description:

> At first our communication was like the pattern that Ruth Middleman describes as "round robin" (Middleman, 1978). We would each take turns talking, going around in a circle. After we had been working together for a while we developed more of a "free floating" communication pattern. Whoever had something to say would just speak out. It was almost as if that person was the leader for that moment. We paid rapt attention to each other–almost hungry for what each other had to say.

Cate, in Group 6, saw her group's interactional pattern reflected in Yalom's diagram of a wheel:

> Yalom offers two diagrams of group interaction–one with the wheel hub and spokes radiating to the rim and the other with interconnections between all the points along the rim (Yalom, 1985). Our group operated on the interconnectedness model rather than the radiating model. The model we used spreads authority and responsibility among all the group members. Each person had the chance to own and share her own authority.

Brown (1991) stresses the interconnectedness between communication and the formation of subgroups. He suggests that subgroups develop through increased communication among group members with common interests. Toseland and Rivas (1984) point out that subgroup formation is a natural and dynamic part of group development. Subgroups become a problem only when the attraction of subgroup members becomes greater than their attraction to the group as a whole.

This problem developed in a number of the student subgroups. It was particularly pronounced in Group 3 where Beth and Caroline, close friends, were embattled with Myra and Sylvie, who formed a strong bond during the course of group development. Marianne, frequently in the scapegoat role, allied at times with Beth and Caroline. Louisa, who loosely allied with the Myra/Sylvie subgroup, also functioned as the mediator between the subgroups. As Beth's log entry reveals, internal group structure greatly influenced the group's communication:

> It is beginning to seem as though all of the real work and meaningful communication for our group takes place apart from official group meetings. The two "power factions" confer as subgroups and bring any decisions back into the larger group. Communication in the larger group mostly takes place between Sylvie, as the leader of her subgroup and me, as the leader of mine. Often, Sylvie and I worked out the major details of an issue while the other group members engaged in cross talk, chit-chatting about something else.

During the course of the semester, Group 3's interactional patterns became increasingly rigid. This culminated, during the group's class presentation, in Louisa literally running from one faction to the other, carrying messages. Louisa describes this complex communication pattern:

> We were in the middle of our presentation, showing the video to the class. Beth and Caroline went out into the hall. Marianne followed them out. During the class break, Beth told me they had decided that we should cut the video short so we did not run out of time. I talked to Sylvie about this and she said absolutely not. We started the video up again and I ran out to the hall to talk to Beth and Caroline (Marianne had appar-

ently left the building altogether). The three of us agreed that the video had to be cut short and I went back into class to tell Sylvie and Myra. I felt like a runner, going back and forth between the two sub-groups. I ended up in a mediator role, talking to each sub-group separately, trying to explain to each group how the other group was feeling about how we should proceed.

GROUP DEVELOPMENT

In most of the groups, students observed a dynamic interplay between the emergence of roles, norms, and interactional patterns and the group's progression through developmental stages. They experienced, first hand, the principle that "a group's entire social structure, its communication and interactional patterns, attraction, social controls, and culture change and evolve as the group develops" (Toseland and Rivas, 1984, p.72).

In several groups, students noted a critical incident in which a member violated a previous norm of not expressing feelings about group process, serving to move the group out of the Power and Control Stage and into the Intimacy Stage (Garland, Jones and Kolodny, 1976). In Group 1 it was Rosie in the role of socio-emotional leader who served this function. The incident, which took place during the fourth meeting, was commented on by all group members but described most vividly by Joan:

When the group meeting started, Rosie jumped right in and expressed anger and frustration about the group process. She did not mince words, saying we are totally stuck in a struggle for power and questioned whether we will ever get past it. She galvanized the group. Everyone began talking at once. I supported Rosie and said I was frustrated too. . . . People talked about how the group process had been uncomfortable for them. Ruth suggested that we rotate the role of facilitator to avoid some of the power struggles.

By the end of the meeting it felt as if the group had finally made some progress. We are not mired anymore, we're on task and finally entering the Intimacy Stage.

A very similar incident took place in the fourth meeting of Group 2 when Barb became angry about being cast in the scapegoat role:

> I was really angry after the third group meeting. I had felt excluded, neglected, scapegoated. It was really painful for me. I knew I had to say something to the group or my anger would cause me to sabotage the group's work. I shared these feelings in the following week's meeting and felt much better. . . .
>
> No one had talked about feelings in the group before, it felt really scary to break this norm but I got a lot of support from the group. Sharing feelings, expressing differences, and mutual support (Yalom, 1985) were normalized. Power and control struggles were minimized thereafter. Some freedom of communication had been established. The group was more cohesive. It was a difficult meeting for me but also an important one. It was a transition into the Intimacy Stage (Garland, Jones, and Kolodny, 1976).

Although not every group experienced such dramatic developmental transitions, the task group experience provided an opportunity to observe some or all of the developmental life span. Serena's summary and analysis of her observations of Group 2 include an overview of the group's passage through the stages of development:

> In the first group meeting we were in the Pre-affiliation Stage. Approach-avoidance behavior was evident between the members, reflecting the lack of clear roles or norms for the group. . . .
>
> We were well into the Power and Control Stage by the third group meeting. The members were jockeying for leadership and some other roles were evident as well (scapegoat, mediator) . . . Issues of rebellion and autonomy surfaced, scapegoating was evident, and cliques began to form for mutual protection.
>
> The fourth meeting saw us move into the Intimacy Stage after Barb expressed her anger and opened up discussion of group process. There was increased responsibility for defining issues, solving problems and working toward constructive solutions. . . .

By the sixth meeting, we had moved into the Differentiation Stage. . . . Group cohesion was very strong. This stage was characterized by freer expression, respect for different opinions, and healthier communication. . . .

We did not actually terminate until our class presentation. We ended with a circle and said good-bye to our group.

STUDENT EVALUATIONS
OF THE TASK GROUP EXPERIENCE

Students evaluated this course assignment in several ways: unsolicited comments in their logs, comments on standardized course evaluation forms and responses on a student self-assessment scale completed at the end of the course. The latter two sources of evaluative data were anonymous. The data suggests that students experienced the task groups as a powerful learning tool. The first comment below is excerpted from a student log, and the second two are responses to the question on the course evaluation form "What has the instructor done that was most helpful?"

Experiencing the group felt like a necessary extension of the readings. It was a great experience to feel the pull and push of the process, the forward and backward motion, the quiet member and the strong leader, all in the same organism.

The task group and log (were most helpful), even though I balked at it initially. It ended up teaching me the most about groups, particularly since I do not have a group at my agency. This assignment really piqued my interest in the readings and made them more relevant—it fit nicely together.

The provision of real life experience with a group was the most helpful to me. . . . Group process became more meaningful—the logs motivated independent inquiry and heightened my awareness of roles and other group dynamics.

Students evaluated their learning from the assignment using a 5-point Likert type scale. The scale was completed by 36 of the 45 students (the remaining nine were unavailable). Students perceived the assignment as increasing their understanding of group roles (89 percent agreed, 67 percent strongly agreed), group norms (94 percent agreed, 72 percent strongly agreed), group interactional patterns (89 percent agreed, 61 percent strongly agreed), and group developmental processes (97 percent agreed, 75 percent strongly agreed). A full 100 percent of students surveyed agreed with the statement ". . . my understanding of group dynamics has increased as a result of my applying them to the group experience."

CONCLUSION

Student task group assignments can effectively utilize "in vivo" learning to foster the application of group theory to practice. Logs provide a vehicle for students to systematically record and examine group processes, applying theoretical constructs to subjective experience (Sullivan and Bibus, 1990). Such "hands-on" classroom learning is particularly important in light of current trends in social work education coupled with decreased opportunities for group experiences in many field settings.

In-class groups clearly cannot take the place of field assignments in developing group facilitation skills. They can, however, function as laboratories for learning about group dynamics. Efforts need to be made to insure that experiential classroom approaches continue to be viewed as supplements to, not substitutes for, field experience.

REFERENCES

Brown, L. (1991). *Groups for growth and change.* New York: Longman.

Garland, J., Jones, H., and Kolodny, R. (1973). A model of stages of group development in social work groups. In S. Bernstein (Ed.). *Explorations in group work practice.* Boston: Milford House, Inc., pp. 17-71.

Latting, J. K. and Raffoul, P. R. (1991). Designing student work groups for increased learning: An empirical investigation. *Journal of Social Work Education*, 27(1): 48-59.

Middleman, R. (1978) Relating group process to group work. *Social Work Practice With Groups*, 1(1): 15-26.

Northen, H. (1988). *Social work with groups.* New York: Columbia University Press.

Radin, N. and Feld, S. (1985). Social psychology for group work practice. In M. Sundel, P. Glasser, R. Sarri, and R. Vintner (Eds.). *Individual change through small groups.* New York: Free Press, pp. 50-69.

Sullivan, M. and Bibus, A. (1990). Discovery of self: One use of logs in graduate school work education. *Journal of Teaching Social Work*, 4(5): 145-157.

Toseland, R. and Rivas, R. (1984). *An introduction to group work practice.* New York: Macmillan.

Yalom, I. (1985). *The theory and practice of group psychotherapy.* New York: Basic Books.

Chapter 7

Social Group Work with Recovering Women: An Empowerment Model

Rita Rhodes
Ann Johnson

The National Institute of Alcohol and Alcohol Abuse (NIAAA) estimates that by 1995, women who have problems with alcohol will number nearly six million (Williams et al., 1987). Despite these numbers, until recently, professionals in the addictions field have not directed their research energies toward women, and as late as 1980, the area was labeled a "nonfield" (Kalant, 1980). In turn, women have not received the proportionate share of resources that their numbers would warrant. Those women who have received treatment were judged to be more abnormal than their male counterparts (Karpman, 1948). The unequal allocation of resources and attention originates, in part, in the failure of addiction models to take into account those factors that shape the experience of female addicts.

MORALITY MODEL

Associated with the temperance movement of the late nineteenth and early twentieth century, was an understanding of alcoholism that linked its etiology to moral failure. This model indicated that moral weakness was the basis of addiction, and improvement in this area was the only satisfactory means to address the problem. As women were considered naturally more moral than men, it followed that the female alcoholic was more deviant in that her addiction went against the natural constraints of feminine morality.

Whereas the moral model is no longer commonly held to be the sole explanatory factor of alcoholism, the linkage between moral laxity and alcoholism remains a popular sentiment. The burden of the stigma is borne by women for whom societal perceptions of alcoholism clash violently with societal images of ideal womanhood. Women stand accused of being unloving mothers and sexually promiscuous (Blume, 1985; Lisansky, 1957). Being more stigmatized than men and ascertained to be more morally defective, women have found their alcoholism treated more as a moral issue than as a health problem.

MEDICAL MODEL

The medical model has provided practitioners and addicted persons alike with a useful framework for understanding problems of addiction from a non-judgmental and non-blaming perspective. Central to the medical model of addiction is the disease concept, formulated in 1960 by a physician, E. M. Jellinek. Identifying alcoholism as a disease was intended to reduce the moral condemnation that had been directed at the addicted (Watts, 1981). The effect, however, was to focus attention on pathology and disease. This way of describing the process of addiction has influenced treatment and sociopolitical processes involved with addictive behavior.

Jellinek's disease model has been adopted by Alcoholics Anonymous and has shaped the treatment delivery system in the field of addiction. The medical model conceptualizes alcoholism as involving an inevitable disease progression that, if unchecked, leads to insanity or death. The etiology of alcoholism stems from a genetic or biological predisposition. In essence, the message of the disease concept is that one does not *develop* alcoholism, but rather that one is *born* an alcoholic.

Members of AA are taught about the disease concept as one way of providing a common culture and framework for recovery. Marty Mann (1975) describes the meaning of the medical model for the recovering alcoholic: "An alcoholic is a very sick person, victim of an insidious, progressive disease, which all too often ends fatally. An alcoholic can be recognized, diagnosed and treated success-fully" (p. 17). Many AA members are convinced that one drink will trigger their compulsion to drink to the point of drunkenness. In some cases, recovering people will talk about inheriting an "alco-holic personality," or a cluster of personality features (such as low frustration tolerance, nervousness or anxiety, codependence, and so forth) which also lead to alcoholism. This inevitability is demon-strated by such statements as "It seems likely that an individual is an alcoholic before he takes his first drink . . . " (Pattison, Sobell, and Sobell, 1977, p. 16). Critical to this understanding is the con-cept of powerlessness that posits that the alcoholic is out of control and unable to exercise any restraint over his or her behavior.

Problems with Medical Model

While providing a non-judgmental discourse for describing alco-hol problems, the medical model posits a linear cause (genetic predisposition) and effect (alcoholism) that does not account for many of the complex features identified with addiction. The role of environmental issues in the transmission of alcoholism is not ad-dressed in a model that limits the sphere of influences and draws the lines of causality too tightly. Multiple influences shape personality and the decisions one makes in choosing a response to the environ-ment. Such complexity is not taken into consideration in a model that depends on an extreme reliance on predisposition. The disease model would be of more service if it were understood as a possible contributing factor to an understanding of addiction rather than as the explanatory model.

Particular Problems with Medical Model for Women

The widespread adoption of the medical model has had important treatment considerations for women. Research and treatment are based on a male experience, and the unique physiological features of female addiction are rarely addressed. Women, for example, are likely to metabolize alcohol differently and smaller quantities can have more adverse effects on their physiology (Gallant, 1990;

Schenker and Speeg, 1990). Because of this overreliance on a male experience, women are interpreted as being "sicker" than male alcoholics when they fail to respond to the interventions that have been based on male clients. In addition, the genetic predisposition that is the basis for the medical model appears less clear in the female experience (Forth-Finegan, 1991).

The medical model, moreover, with its linear cause and effect explanation does not adequately account for many of the complex features identified with female addiction. Factors such as family, socioeconomics, education, wage earning potential, personal and social skills, victimization, and adult relationships are deeply embedded in the lives of women. The role of environmental issues in the transmission of alcoholism is difficult to assess. What does appear to be true is that women are at significant risk for the development of alcoholism because of their vulnerable roles in the larger society.

Victimization

One of the shared vulnerabilities among women alcoholics and addicts is an experience with victimization and abuse. Estimates of the prevalence of victimization among recovering women range from 12 percent to 74 percent (Beckman, 1984; Lindberg and Distad, 1985; Rohsenow, Corbett, and Devine, 1988; Wilsnack, 1984). One study described the population of female incest victims as having drug abuse rates that were seven times higher than those of other women (Peluso and Peluso, 1988). Women traditionally have not been treated sympathetically; victim-blaming is common practice, with the most recent example being the practice of criminalizing pregnant substance abusers under the guise of child protection laws. Given societal responses and women's corresponding internalization of the shame that is created by the abuse, the development of female addictive behaviors seems more a response to environmental rather than personal causes.

Depression

Female addicts are also more likely to share a background that includes an experience of clinical depression and other mental illnesses than are their male counterparts (Gomberg and Lisansky, 1984; Schuckit, 1986; Turnbull and Gomberg, 1988). Women alcoholics, moreover, have lower self-esteem than other women or male alcoholics (Braiker, 1984). Given the numerical domination of women among the clinically depressed, it is not inconsistent that female addicts would present with a history of depression when entering into treatment (Blume, 1985). Given the preponderance of depression among women and the growing literature that describes the linkage between depression and addictive behaviors, it appears that an overreliance upon a medical model to explain female addiction leaves out significant environmental factors that might explain the depression as well as the addiction (Van Den Bergh, 1991). Factors such as abuse, poverty, educational disadvantages, and responsibility for young children have been identified as placing women at risk for depression as well as addiction (Gomberg and Lisansky, 1984; Lewinsohn, Hoberman, and Rosenbaum, 1988; McGrath, Keita, Strickland, and Russo, 1990; Stoppard, 1989).

ECOLOGICAL MODEL

Thus, it seems safe to conclude that the medical model alone fails to provide a very complete understanding of the female addict. Whereas the medical model is useful in providing unbiased language with which to describe the alcoholic woman, it provides a disservice as well. For women in particular, a more complex systems approach is most likely to take into account the many factors that come into play in female addiction. An ecological model of causation, which places the person within her environment, offers a more robust model for describing the addictive process and its effect on women.

A further advantage of the ecological model for treating alcoholic women is its more comprehensive descriptions of success. In AA, an alcoholic is either sober or not. It is this either/or dichotomy that makes success more difficult to attain. The ecological model, which ascribes to the public health model of moving on a continuum from disease to wellness, allows for incremental growth and varying perceptions of success and growth. The AA model sets up women for failure when they cannot stay abstinent. This overlooks the possibility that it might be possible for a woman to end an abusive relationship, a success for her, or to make a vocational change, which gives her more income, and be able to acknowledge these successes.

In addition, an ecological understanding of female addictions suggests interventions. "The ecological model portrays multiple causal influences and any instance of disease is seen as the result of reciprocal interactions of several factors. The factors themselves—agent, host, and environment, or rather, specific variables associated with each—are perhaps best not viewed as "causes" but as concepts incorporated in descriptions of ecological relationships" (Kane, 1981, p. 68). By enlarging our sphere of causation, we are then able to address treatment concerns from a multifaceted approach. Such a broadbased understanding of etiology points out the direction for effective intervention.

We are arguing that a broadbased understanding of female addiction is critical for creating effective interventions. The disease model with a single unit of causation implies a treatment focus primarily aimed at changing the thinking of the alcoholic (12 steps of AA). The ecological model, with a dynamic interplay of causation, implies change in the person as well as the environment, and in the way the alcoholic woman interacts with her environment. The complexities of the issues that cause and support female addiction are revealed in a list of treatment issues developed by Norma Finkelstein, Director of the Coalition on Addiction, Pregnancy and Parenting in Cambridge, Massachusetts. These include:

1. guilt, stigma, shame;
2. sexualized image—"whore" and "slut";
3. low self-esteem;
4. feelings of powerlessness and learned helplessness;
5. relationships in women's lives;
6. care and needs of children;
7. family violence, sexual abuse, and incest;
8. AIDS;
9. multiple addictions;
10. vocational and economic issues;
11. drinking, drugging, and pregnancy;

12. anger and depression;
13. eating disorders;
14. physiological considerations (1990, p 22).

A number of the issues on this list are social problems, not personal ones.

AN EMPOWERMENT MODEL OF GROUP WORK

The concept of powerlessness, so central to the teachings of the medical model, serves women ill, because it is essentially that very feeling, powerlessness, that characterizes the lives of so many women. The present approach to addictions treatment may, in fact, be disempowering. According to James Sandel (1990), counselors frequently advise clients to "do it because it works" and to "let us do your thinking for you," as they introduce the 12-step program (p. 34). Rather than strengthen the client's own thinking abilities, this approach may actually diminish a woman's ability to make thoughtful decisions in her own self-interest. Recovery begins for women when they begin to feel empowered.

The purpose of our group intervention is not primarily to organize broadbased community interventions to make sweeping changes in the culture (which in subtle and not so subtle ways supports abuse to women), although it might be useful for this to occur. Rather, the goal of the group empowerment model is to help alcoholic women acquire the skills they need to negotiate successfully the environment on personal, vocational, political, and interrelational levels. In order to accomplish this goal, we need "to empower clients, to teach them that the needed abilities and resources are found within." An empowerment model would serve to "create a safe environment to assist the client in permitting attitudinal, behavioral, or belief changes to occur at a rate that is comfortable and appropriate" (Orman, 1990, p. 8). The issue of empowerment is particularly a difficult issue for recovering women who are often more comfortable with admitting their powerlessness than with accepting the real power that they are capable of exerting in their lives. An empowerment model encourages women to take responsibility for making things happen in their lives while acknowledging the real barriers that present obstacles to such overtures. It also encourages women to take credit and acknowledge their achievements rather than dismiss them as unimportant or as the work of others (Van Den Bergh, 1991).

An empowerment model of group work differs from a psychotherapeutic model in that learning focuses on the here and now rather than on psychodynamic processes. In an empowerment model, the entire focus is not personal. There are group goals as well as individual goals. Group goals relate to the social situation in which women find themselves and their problem solving skills in dealing with the social milieu.

CRISIS WORK

The uses of group work for empowerment purposes need to be separated from what is essentially crisis intervention. When women first enter treatment for addictions, they are likely to be in crisis. Whereas men enter treatment programs after years of disruptive drinking, women are more likely to be propelled into treatment following a significant life crisis such as a divorce, the death of a child, a significant medical emergency, or traumatization from violence such as rape or spousal abuse. The primary order of business is to help her through the crisis while maintaining abstinence in a supportive atmosphere. Only after a period of physical and emotional stabilization can the female alcoholic begin to acquire new approaches to dealing with problems. The kind of group experience we are recommending for long-term therapeutic gains is an outpatient experience that begins after some period of sobriety has been established and that is not crisis focused. It is recommended that members have a minimum of ninety days of sobriety (Orosz, 1982).

VALUE OF GROUP EXPERIENCE
FOR WOMEN

There are a number of cogent reasons why group therapy is the ideal model of treatment for recovering clients. As far back as 1946 when Kurt Lewin began human relations training to deal with the tensions of race relations, it became apparent that experiential learning–observing one's own behavior and its effect on others–was a powerful tool for change (Yalom, 1975, p. 460). In addition, alcoholics tend to develop a complex system of denial that protects them from the reality of their situation. The recognition of common patterns, the opportunity for gentle confrontation, and the commonalties of thought patterns, all are best addressed in a group situation.

For women, moreover, the experience of recovery is a lonely struggle of feeling "different" and out of focus. Incorporating feelings of worthlessness into their self-images, many recovering women may feel hopeless and depressed. One clear advantage of a group intervention is in overcoming alienation. The experiences of one recovering woman when added to those of others illuminate the notion that women as a class are victimized. The solutions to a woman's problems are not all personal but can be found also in ameliorating the forces in society that deprive women of power. The personal becomes the political; and this transformation in the recovering woman's thinking is essential for her to become empowered. It is important for women to abandon the notion that it is "all their fault." Lastly, the sharing of common experiences lends itself to the discovery that the commonality women share is a societal position that fails to address the needs of women.

CONTENT

This chapter will identify the major concepts that we have utilized with recovering women in an outpatient setting. These include problem solving, feelings, relationships, and parenting. It will include a discussion of how each concept is particularly relevant for women and their struggle with recovery. Finally, it will discuss how these concepts are used to expand the power that women have over their lives.

Problem Solving

Given the overall goal of empowerment, it is useful to teach recovering women the concept of problem solving. In the model that we employ, women are taught not only a problem-solving approach, but also an awareness of the feelings associated with the problem. The teaching of this skill lends itself to the group process where there is real therapeutic value attached to the sharing of problems with others in a similar situation. Group members are both creative in supplying possible solutions to identified problems and realistic about the consequences associated with certain choices. The women are most helpful to each other when trust has been established and they are able to share their concerns and responses to such problems as employment, housing, health, and ongoing sobriety. These are problems that are unlikely to be shared in other settings, and the solutions that are developed can have an immediate impact on the women's lives. Such practices are effective in helping women develop an internal locus of control, which, in turn, works to increase self-esteem.

We believe that a knowledge of the problem-solving process encourages women to develop an awareness of the areas for choice in their lives. We hope to promote an understanding that women have a right to make choices that contribute to their safety and wellbeing and encourage an attitude that it is good self-care to ask for help. In addition, we want to expand the world that these women inhabit and affirm that they are not alone and that there are people who can help them.

Feelings Work

In alcoholic families, individuals learn to distrust their own feelings by familial behavior that denies or ignores their emotional response to the environment. Given this history, addicted adults often numb or deny feelings by means of chemicals or other addictive behaviors. For recovering clients, an awareness of feelings, as well as their expression, is new and uncomfortable behavior. Our group provides clients with exercises by which they can learn to begin to trust their feelings and claim ownership of them. The use of "I" statements is modeled. Group membership supports the expression of common emotions that individuals previously believed were unique to their experience. Such participation helps women to trust their feelings, which also promotes a sense of empowerment.

As women move into recovery, anger is an emotion that causes a great deal of anxiety. Women, in general, have not been socialized to express anger and seem more comfortable with suppressing this emotion. Along with education about the need to express all emotions safely, particular exercises and role playing that encourage the expression of anger are identified. We educate clients to the idea that they have a right to their anger and about the relationship between repressed anger and depression. We use programmatic activities that demonstrate the problems that stem from the repression of feelings and emphasize the unhealthy consequences of such a regular practice. For recovering women, who are likely to have a history of abuse, activities would demonstrate that the energy associated with anger can be utilized for the accomplishment of goals (Van den Bergh, 1991).

Relationships

The role of relationships in the recovery efforts of women is critical. For recovering women, dependency issues involving chemicals are frequently coupled with dependency issues around relationships. The group experience offers women the opportunity to examine the role that they play in relationships and the extent to which they rely on others to provide meaning and purpose in life (Van Den Bergh, 1991). Dependency issues are explored and activities are directed toward getting women to take responsibility for their own well being. Assertiveness training is introduced to help women learn to identify needs and make requests.

The group also encourages women to explore "a way of being with others that allows her also to be with herself" (Gilligan, 1982, p. 53). Women are socialized to be caretakers, and this orientation is particularly problematic for females in recovery. In the struggle to juggle the demands of family and the demands of recovery, the balance is likely to be weighted in favor of the former. The concept of selfishness has particular meaning for recovering women who frequently interpret expectations for the expenditure of time and energy on personal recovery as selfish endeavors. The group experience is useful in helping women create a hierarchy of needs that does not routinely sacrifice their own recovery to the needs of others.

Parenting

Probably no other issue contributes to the pain of recovery for women more than their behavior toward their children when they were drinking. Since so much of feminine identity is associated with the role of motherhood, recovering women feel enormous shame around their failure to parent successfully. The group experience is powerful in permitting women to relate behavior that is shameful for them in an accepting environment. Such an environment also promotes a forgiveness of self for not knowing how to parent. Such forgiveness promotes empowerment, which itself is the basis for future successful parenting.

Related to the painful memories, associated with their parenting when they were drinking, is the confusion that women experience in these parent/child relationships in their sobriety. So many of their expectations, as well as their children's expectations, were shaped by fantasies of recovery, that the letdown and confusion are almost as painful as the earlier drinking behavior. The group experience is helpful when women hear that they are not alone in struggling with parenting issues while attempting to maintain recovery. Educational efforts focus on helping participants learn new ways to relate to children.

Evaluation of Outcome

Too frequently the criterion for successful treatment completion is total abstinence from alcohol and adherence to a 12-step program. The ecological model, while recognizing the health-enhancing consequences of abstinence for recovering women, also recognizes gains in other areas of life. Because the term *empowerment* is somewhat abstract, it is difficult to measure with any degree of accuracy. More concrete indicators can be identified that are attributes of empowerment. Some of these might include an increase in earnings, level of educational attainment, access to medical care (ongoing preventative medical care, not just emergency care), reduction in home accidents, or in battering incidents, control over conception, absence of physical disease, knowledge of resources available in community, ability to make financial decisions and manage money (knowing how to establish credit, apply for a loan, file income taxes, etc.), and satisfaction with relationships. These indicators can be identified with a good deal of precision. They recognize that circumstances of life are dynamic and interactive and can influence each other in sometimes surprising and unexpected ways. One drink does not cancel out other gains and does not have to be perceived as treatment failure. The value of the model is that wellness or recovery does not occur as an either/or dichotomy, but as progress along a continuum from disease to well-being.

IMPLICATIONS FOR SOCIAL WORK PRACTICE

A systemic view of addictions is not only a useful way of understanding female addiction but is consistent with effective social work practice. Such an understanding, we believe, places the social work profession with its interest in the transactions between individuals and their environments as the logical profession to address the needs of female addicts. The intervention that such an understanding promotes, a group empowerment model, is also consistent with the roots of social work practice that sought to organize people to act on their own behalf. The goal of empowerment, moreover, is also related to the social work orientation of identifying strengths.

We also believe that effective intervention in addictions issues is promoted by effective assessment. Whereas a medical model of alcoholism assumes one prescription and standardized treatment, an ecological perspective takes into account the complexity of systems that are involved in sustaining the addiction. The medical model is premised on the male experience and is particularly inappropriate for understanding female addiction. A systems approach to addictions does not exclude a disease component in an addictions model, but it avoids the oversimplification that is particularly damaging to promoting successful interventions on behalf of female addicts. Rigorous training in the varying systems involved in assessment is the best guarantee that social workers will successfully serve their female clients who are in recovery.

REFERENCES

Beckman, L. J. (1984). Treatment needs of women alcoholics. *Alcoholism Treatment Quarterly, 1*, 101-114.

Blume, S. B. (1985). Women and Alcohol. In T. E. Bratter and G. G. Forrest (Eds.). *Alcoholism and substance abuse* (pp. 623-638). New York: The Free Press.

Braiker, H. (1984). Therapeutic issues in the treatment of alcoholic women. In S. Wilsnack and L. Beckman (Eds.). *Alcohol problems in women* (pp. 349-368). New York: The Guilford Press.

Finkelstein, N. (1990). Changing needs of today's addicted women. *Counselor Magazine, 8*, 21-23.

Forth-Finegan, J. L. (1991). Sugar and spice and everything nice: Gender socialization and women's addiction–a literature review. In C. Bepko (Ed.). *Feminism and addiction* (pp. 19-48). New York: The Haworth Press.

Gallant, D. M. (1990). Female alcohol abusers: Vulnerability to multiple organ damage. *Alcohol: Clinical and Experimental Research, 14(2)*, 260.

Gilligan, C. (1982). *In a different voice: Psychological theory and women's development.* Cambridge, MA: Harvard University Press.

Gomberg, E. and Lisansky, J. (1984). Antecedents of alcohol problems in women. In S. Wilsnack and L. Beckman (Eds.). *Alcohol problems in women* (pp. 233-259). New York: The Guilford Press.

Jellinek, E. M. (1960). *The disease concept of alcoholism.* New Haven: College and University Press.

Kalant, O. J. (1980) (Ed.). *Research advances in alcohol and drug problems. (Vol. 5: Alcohol and drug problems in women).* New York: Plenum.

Kane, G. (1981). *Inner city alcoholism.* New York: Human Science Press.

Karpman, B. M. (1948). *The alcoholic woman.* Washington, DC: Linacre.

Lewinsohn, P. M., Hoberman, H., and Rosenbaum, M. (1988). A prospective study of the risk factors for unipolar depression. *Journal of Abnormal Psychology, 97*, 251-264.

Lindberg, F. H. and Distad, L. J. (1985). Post-traumatic stress disorders in women who experienced childhood incest. *Child Abuse and Neglect, 9*, 329-334.

Lisansky, E. S. (1957). Alcoholism in women: Social and psychological concomitants. *Quarterly Journal of Studies on Alcohol, 18*, 588-623.

Mann, M. (1975). *New primer on alcoholism.* New York: Holt, Rinehart, and Winston.

McGrath, E., Keita, G., Strickland, B., and Russo, N. (1990). *Women and depression: Risk factors and treatment issues.* Washington, DC: American Psychological Association.

Orman, D. (1990). The myth of the ACOA. *Counselor Magazine, 8*, 8, 46.

Orosz, S. B. (1982). Assertiveness in recovery. *Social Work with Groups, 5*, 25-31.

Pattison, E. M., Sobell, M., and Sobell, L. (1977). *Emerging concepts of alcohol dependence.* New York: Springer.

Peluso, E. and Peluso L. (1988). *Women and drugs: Getting hooked, getting clean.* Minneapolis: Compucare.

Rohsenow, D. J., Corbett, R., and Devine, D. (1988). Molested as children: A hidden contribution to substance abuse? *Journal of Substance Abuse Treatment, 5*, 13-18.

Sandel, J. (1990). From self to self: Making recovery real. *Counselor Magazine, 8*, 34-37.

Schenker, S. and Speeg, K. V. (1990). The risk of alcohol intake in men and women: All may not be equal. *New England Journal of Medicine, 322*, 127-129.

Schuckit, M. (1986). Genetic and clinical implications of alcoholism and affective disorders. *American Journal of Psychiatry, 143*, 140-147.

Stoppard, J. M. (1989). An evaluation of cognitive/behavioral theories for understanding depression in women. *Canadian Psychology, 30*, 39-47.

Turnbull, J. E. and Gomberg, E. S. L. (1988). Impact of depressive symptomatology on alcohol problems in women. *Alcoholism: Clinical and Experimental Research, 12*, 371-381.

Van Den Bergh, N. (1991). Having bitten the apple: A feminist perspective on addictions. In N. Van Den Bergh (Ed.). *Feminist perspectives on addictions* (pp. 330). New York: Springer Publishing Co., Inc.

Williams, G. D., Stinson, F. S., Parker, D. A., Harford, T. C., and Noble, J. (1987). Epidemiological Bulletin No. 15: Demographic trends, alcohol abuse and alcoholism 1985-1995. *Alcohol Health and Research World, 11*, 80-83.

Wilsnack, S. (1984). Drinking, sexuality and sexual dysfunction in women. In S. Wilsnack and L. Beckman (Eds.). *Alcohol problems in women* (pp. 189-227). New York: The Guilford Press.

Yalom, I. (1975). *The theory and practice of group psychotherapy.* New York: Basic Books.

Chapter 8

Redefining Adult Identity: A Coming Out Group for Lesbians

Anna Travers

LESBIANS, HOMOPHOBIA, AND THE COMING OUT PROCESS

Lesbians experience severe personal, familial, institutional, and legal restrictions to full or equal participation in society and a lack of protection against discrimination on the basis of their sexual identity. Historically, homosexual behavior has been regarded as sinful, sick or, in the case of lesbians, nonexistent or invisible. Even today, while liberal humanists assert greater tolerance for "alternative lifestyles," the fact that lesbians and gays are still rejected by their families, fired from jobs, denied spousal rights and benefits, deemed unfit parents in divorce, adoption, and foster care situations, denied proper medical care, turned down as immigrants, and harassed and assaulted on a daily basis refutes the reality of this claim. Individual and systemic homophobia is perpetuated through these sanctions that serve to limit the validity and expression of lesbian and gay sexual identities.

Likewise, the socialization of young people into adult sexuality focuses entirely on heterosexuality, with homosexuality being ignored or discussed in pejorative and usually inaccurate ways. It is normative for everyone to adopt a heterosexual identity and heterosexual behavior and to actively discount, resist, and fear same sex attractions and relationships. Individuals who eventually identify as lesbian or gay have to go through a process of recognizing thoughts, feelings, and/or behaviors that place them at odds with the social and cultural norms governing intimate relationships.

For lesbians, the initial questioning of heterosexual identification may come about in a variety of ways: there may be a recognition that sexual attraction has always been directed toward other women; there may be a shift away from a heterosexual identity as a result of increasing intimacy with women, in general, or an involvement with a particular woman; or, for some feminists, the decision to identify as a lesbian may reflect a political choice to limit primary relationships to other women. Regardless of how the split from normative heterosexual identity comes about, women who are coming out begin a process of exploring and defining the meaning of this change in sexual identity, and considering its implications in every significant area of their lives.

The change to a lesbian identity not only represents an explicit relational shift in terms of primary emotional and sexual partners, it also represents a downward shift in social acceptability, and this is the root of the existential crisis that many women experience. In Erving Goffman's terminology, homosexuals become part of the "discreditable," "whose stigma is not apparent from appearance but due to a "failing" which is not usually apparent until the person reveals it" (Goffman, 1963, p. 62). The nature of this "failing" is rarely discussed in the literature, however, even in the extensive literature that has emerged around the psychology and mental health of gays and lesbians. Where once homosexuality itself was the problem, now homophobia–the irrational fear and hatred of homosexuals–is constantly acknowledged as *the central issue* affecting lesbians and gays. And yet an analysis of homophobia and its function in society is rarely part of the frame of reference or the explicit work of mental health practitioners. Theorists and therapists alike focus on the psychological aspects of prejudice without reference to its social or political roots. Feminist scholars, such as Marilyn Frye (1980) and Sheila Jeffreys (1990), note that this failure to contextualize homophobia results in a baffling tendency to deny its impact or even to blame the victim. Suzanne Pharr (1988) explains lesbian oppression thus: "To be a lesbian is to be perceived as someone who has stepped out of line, who has moved out of sexual/economic dependence on a male, who is woman identified. . . . A lesbian is perceived as a threat to the nuclear family, to male domi-nance and control, to the very heart of sexism" (Pharr, 1988, p. 18).

Viewed in this light, lesbianism is not merely an "alternative lifestyle" within the patriarchal system but a potential alternative to the patriarchal system, and therein lies its threat and its promise. This is not to say that all lesbians consciously regard their lives in this way, but intuitively lesbians know they are in some sense "out of bounds" and at the same time "home safe." This paradox has been a major focus of lesbian culture, politics, academic study, and everyday life (Rich, 1980; Frye, 1980; Lorde, 1987).

For practitioners working with women who are coming out as lesbians, it is important to validate the complexities and contradic-tions inherent in lesbian existence and, at the same time, to provide mechanisms for the development of community support and indi-vidual integrity. Group work can be an ideal way of accomplishing these multiple goals in a safe and positive environment.

IDENTITY ISSUES FOR LESBIANS WHO ARE COMING OUT

The concept of redefining adult identity recognizes the fact that lesbians frequently come out once they are mature adults. Various researchers have used the notion of identity development to explain the cognitive, affective, and behavioral dimensions of the coming out process and to describe a common sequence of stages. Most models of the coming out process (Cass, 1979; Coleman, 1982) describe a hierarchical developmental model of identity formation, in which the gay or lesbian person moves from identity confusion to first relationships, disclosure to significant others, involvement in the gay or lesbian community, and ultimately to "integration" where being lesbian or gay is no longer so important and is bal-anced with other identities. Critics of these models, for example, Celia Kitzinger, object to the notion that being politically active in the struggle against homophobia represents the penultimate step in reaching true maturity, and note that "intervention is overwhelm-ingly focused on person-change rather than system-change, i.e., helping the individual achieve self-fulfillment and personal happi-ness in a homophobic world." (Kitzinger, 1987, p. 39)

In fact, there is general agreement that women will go through different aspects of the coming out process in different sequences based on issues such as economics, family norms, religion, and access to the lesbian community. It may, therefore, be useful to recognize the multi-dimensional nature of the coming out process in terms of stages. Individuals cope, in reality, not as a linear progression, but in a feedback loop in which personal actions or disclosures lead to societal responses that, in turn, affect the person's subsequent actions and modify a developing sense of self (de Monteflores and Schultz, 1978).

Whatever the order in which women tackle the many tasks of coming out as lesbians, they are almost certain to face difficult decisions and an emotionally turbulent period in their lives (Loewenstein, 1980). First, they often feel extremely isolated as they experience the loss of heterosexual privilege (become one of the discreditable), begin to feel the split between public and private life, and have yet to develop friends and connections in the lesbian community. Internally, there is frequently a sense of being bad, weird, or shameful as women confront their own internalized homophobia and beliefs regarding sexual orientation, gender, and sex roles.

Relationships with family members and friends frequently become strained, either because women feel they can no longer talk about important issues or because they anticipate hostility or rejection if they disclose their lesbianism (Zitter, 1987). Even where disclosures have not been disastrous, there is often denial, disappointment, or distancing that removes the very support system that most people turn to when undergoing a personal crisis. This fact then increases isolation and self blame.

Identity is also closely tied to membership in broader social, cultural, racial, or religious groups (ties that may be crucial for survival in some oppressed groups), but these too will have to be examined and possibly renegotiated. This may create tremendous conflicts of loyalty and personal integrity as women must choose between belonging to one community or another (Lorde, 1987; Espin, 1987).

Expectations of the future, such as long-term coupling, parenthood, and economic security, may again become issues for women who, as adults, may have defined or been perceived to have defined their goals and life plans from a heterosexual perspective. For some women, the shift to a lesbian identity may involve ending a marriage, losing a home, and actually or potentially losing their children. For such women, experiences of loss and "being lost" can be intense.

At the same time, and this can be confusing, women who are coming out frequently experience powerful positive feelings as they make sense of their "differentness" and acknowledge their need for primary relationships with other women. Many experience a feeling of relief and wholeness. Others view existing or potential relationships with a sense of joy, excitement, or sexual fulfillment. For some women, lesbianism is consistent with or may be an outcome of their feminist politics and, for these women in particular, identifying as a lesbian may hold the promise of a radical alternative to patriarchal models of relationship and community.

THE APPROPRIATENESS OF GROUP WORK

The choice of group work rather than individual counseling reflects the belief that most women who are coming out as lesbians do not need therapy, and that a group is the most appropriate way to deal with both a major identity shift and a loss of social status. The approach used incorporates much of the theory and methodology of social group work, which has its roots in the settlement and neighborhood houses of poor and immigrant populations, and combines it with more recently developed feminist social work practice. Key features from each perspective will be illustrated, and the overlap and differences between the two will be discussed.

Ruth Middleman, a noted social group work theorist, asserts that group process itself has been shown to be a powerful change dynamic, creating a micro-society in which individuals can safely explore and try out new roles in an atmosphere of mutual support (Middleman and Goldberg, 1988). Many of the women in the coming out group had never before talked to more than one or two lesbians; they were unsure about how to identify themselves and how to interact. For socially oppressed and isolated populations, in particular, the group process can counteract internalized negative feelings about the self. In Gitterman's words "As members experience continuing support, they are likely to risk more personal, even taboo concerns. This process itself helps members to experience their concerns and problems as being less private and deviant. [It] reduces isolation, 'depathologises' problems and diminishes stigma" (Gitterman, 1989).

Again reflecting social group work method, the goals of the Women's Coming Out Group were multiple, addressing a combination of the personal and social functioning needs of its members (Alissi, 1981). Different members had different priorities, but the goals reflected a cluster of cognitive, emotional, practical, and social concerns common to lesbians at the beginning of the coming out process.

1. To help women become more clear and comfortable in defining their sexual orientation.
2. To explore and alleviate feelings of conflict and distress.
3. To provide mutual aid around common problems and decisions.
4. To become more familiar with the lesbian community and reduce isolation.

In order to achieve the last goal of becoming more familiar with the lesbian community and reducing isolation, the group members were encouraged to socialize with each other and to participate in lesbian cultural and leisure activities together. As Glassman and Kates advocate, "The group itself is taken as a natural part of a larger whole and is to be worked within that context whenever possible" (Glassman and Kates, 1990, p. 16). For the women in the Coming Out Group, this parallel, autonomous contact became a feature of every group within the first few weeks. It intensified both the development of group process and the ability of individuals to create new social identities. At least one of the groups continues to meet socially two years later and other members have formed lasting friendships.

Over the past two or three decades, feminists have used groups extensively for consciousness raising, problem solving, and political organizing, often combining all three elements together. Feminist practice has incorporated some of the traditional principles and values of social group work, such as building on strengths, the validation and support of every member, the development of mutual aid and democratic process. But feminism has parted company with the more neutral or conservative perspectives inherent in systems theory or ecological models that underpin most social group work. Elizabeth Lewis describes the difference thus: "Feminist perspectives, on the other hand, require the capacity to critique the system, to deconstruct it in its own essentially discriminatory aspects and to call by name those attitudes and expectations, terms of language, behaviors and social arrangements which cumulatively, have a disadvantaging, marginalizing effect" (Lewis, 1987, p. 11).

Feminist analysis has produced paradigms and methodologies that can be applied not only to issues of gender inequality, but to other forms of discrimination and oppression such as racism, classism, heterosexism, ageism, able-ism, etc. In fact, there is increasing interest in integrated models of analysis and practice where the combined effect of various kinds of discrimination can be understood and addressed. (Pharr, 1988; Fulani, 1987)

Group work provides a natural forum in which to explore critically the social construction of concepts such as gender, sex roles, sexuality, race, and culture using everyday language and the collective history and experiences of the members. Kitzinger explains this radical feminist perspective thus: "Central to this argument is the assumption that our 'inner selves'—the way we think and feel about and how we define ourselves—are connected in an active and reciprocal way with the larger social and political structures and processes in the context of which they are constructed" (Kitzinger, 1987, p. 62). An existential crisis, like coming out as a lesbian, will almost inevitably raise questions about what is natural or acceptable in human nature and social relations. A group can provide the opportunity and support for women who are coming out to challenge a social system that tells them they are unacceptable and to counteract the negative stereotyping that can corrode self-image and social competence. Topics chosen by the group, such as understanding and dealing with homophobia, lesbian sexuality, relationships, and community all lent themselves to discussion of the accepted meanings of these concepts and the possibility of defining and creating new and more appropriate ones.

COMPOSITION OF THE GROUP

The Coming Out Group for Women was developed and led by the author, a lesbian social worker with a background in group work, at the Toronto Counselling Centre for Lesbians and Gays. Leadership by an openly lesbian worker in a lesbian/gay-run agency clearly gave a message of community support and pride that was generally appreciated by the members. It helped to depathologize both lesbianism and the coming out process while providing an atmosphere of empathy and respect. For a few women, even entering an organization run by lesbians and gays caused additional anxiety at first, but this was soon overcome.

The group was offered three times, for ten weeks each, during a one-year period. All prospective group members participated in an individual meeting with the worker to ensure that at least some of the proposed goals were in line with their needs and to receive more information about the group. In addition, other issues such as alcohol or drug problems, eating disorders, sexual or physical abuse, and experiences of racism, poverty, or war were explored. This information enabled the worker to discuss with some women the need for other services or supports and to clarify the areas that could be dealt with in the group. It was important to set out these boundaries from the beginning as group membership was intended to be as inclusive as possible, but, since the group leader was a volunteer with a full-time job, the opportunities for individual support were limited.

As it turned out, most of the women were already seeing a counselor or therapist, and the majority reported stress-related phenomena such as depression, anxiety, chronic headaches, and mood swings. Most women attributed these problems to confusion and pain about their sexual orientation. About one quarter of the women also reported more severe emotional difficulties including alcohol abuse, anorexia, severe depression, suicide attempts, and self-mutilation. All these women with more serious difficulties had histories of emotional, physical, or sexual abuse. Some had been helped in dealing with these issues, others had not or had been further victimized by the psychiatric system.

The thirty or so group members who participated in the three groups ranged in age from 19 to 42. This wide age range presented some difficulty, especially for the the two or three older members who were vastly outnumbered by members in their twenties. These older women worried that they would not have enough in common with the younger members and that the kinds of life decisions they were facing would be different. Two of them did remain involved, however, and found the group rewarding while a third member dropped out.

Almost all the women in the coming out groups were working or were students. The occupations listed by the members included retail clerk, nurse, researcher, artist, claims adjuster, librarian, broadcaster, former nun, teacher, receptionist, and film technician. One woman lived on government assistance due to physical and emotional difficulties, another was supported by her husband and never left the apartment alone, and another was a part-time student and the mother of two small children.

The majority of the women were white and had been born in Canada, two were black or of mixed racial background, one was Chinese and one was part Native Canadian. Most women were fairly new to Toronto, having grown up in other parts of Canada, often in small towns or rural areas. Many had come to the city to obtain jobs or education, some were seeking an escape from small-town prejudice, and most reported feeling isolated and lonely.

GROUP STRUCTURE AND CONTENT

The approach used in the Women's Coming Out Group combined topic areas chosen by the group members with activities and exercises designed by the facilitator. Structured programming was used to encourage high levels of participation and to deepen the level of group discussion in a group that was of fairly short duration (ten weeks). Check-ins at the beginning of the sessions allowed the group to be aware of important events that had happened to members during the week; and check-outs at the end enabled the group to discuss the impact of the session and to review the group process.

As mentioned earlier, group members were also encouraged to meet on their own between sessions and to participate in activities in the community. The only restriction was that members were asked not to enter into sexual relationships until after the group ended as it was felt that this might lead to problematic group dynamics.

The first session was designed to give group members a chance to meet each other in a non-stressful way, to clarify expectations, and to set ground rules. Generally speaking, the members were extremely anxious about coming to the group, and so most of the introductory activities took place in pairs and groups of three or four. Due to the fears involved in the coming out process, two issues of particular importance emerged. A discussion of confidentiality included how members should acknowledge each other if they met outside the group, how information could identify a person even if their name was not used, and an understanding that confidentiality meant "forever." Another key concern was that the goal of the group should not be to "make everyone be a lesbian." Although this had *not* been stated as one of the initial goals, it was important to reiterate that becoming more clear about sexual orientation and less confused or distressed did not mean that any woman had to adopt any particular label.

The second and third sessions of the group were devoted to the sharing of individual stories about growing up as a sexual person. Members were invited to tell their story in their own words or to use a simple set of questions that traced awareness of early sexual feelings, attractions, and experiences in childhood and adolescence, and adult emotional and sexual relationships. The questions included attractions and experiences with either men or women and did not imply any particular causal factors with regard to sexual orientation. The group leader also told her coming out story, emphasizing both the struggles she shared with the other women and also the possibility of establishing a sense of wholeness and purpose.

Because most lesbians have spent much of their energy minimizing, denying, forgetting, or being silent about their attractions to or involvements with other women, reclaiming and telling their own sexual histories provided the members with a way of integrating these "lost" elements and seeing the threads that had led them to this point. By talking in the group, the women also received validation and acceptance from others and began to feel more connected. Finally, the sharing of individual stories pointed to various common themes and experiences that were reflected in the topics chosen for later sessions. Members found the activity fairly stressful, but agreed that it was important to do it. Most women felt "excited" and "high" after the sessions; a few reacted with tears and anger because they "felt they had wasted so much of their lives."

At the end of the third session, the members chose a series of topics for the remainder of the group. In all three groups, the topics were fairly consistent and usually included the following:

- Coming out to family and friends
- Understanding and dealing with homophobia
- Dating and relationships
- Lesbian sexuality
- The lesbian community
- Planning for the future
- Evaluation and celebration

Discussions about religion, racial and cultural ties, and having children, also came up spontaneously in most of the groups. Due to the constraints of this chapter there is only space to describe a few of the topics and to illustrate some group dynamics that may be particular to this type of group.

The topic of understanding and dealing with homophobia was one in which it seemed essential to try to move outside the circle of discrimination and self-hatred. Using the women's individual life histories, the group examined the beliefs about gays and lesbians that they had learned growing up. Not only were the "messages" very negative, but they were full of myths about child abusers, uncontrolled sex fiends, women with beards, etc. The group then discussed whether these images corresponded with their experiences of themselves or other lesbians they knew.

The members then used the same process to examine their socialization as girls and the expectations of them as women. Almost all reported that marriage and motherhood were key values, whatever other aspirations may have been encouraged. As the discussion progressed, the members were able to look at the ways in which, as lesbians, they might fail to fulfill traditional female role expectations. The link in traditional value systems between heterosexual relationships, sex roles, and womanhood itself was a concept that many women were familiar with already, but by pairing this discussion with the other about lesbians, the members were able to understand some of the underlying reasons for feeling bad and ashamed. As one group member said "We break all the rules, don't we." It was an emotional session and, like many, it led to relief for some and a deepening of anxieties for others.

The session on coming out to family and friends was another pressing issue for most of the members. Although many felt alienated by their secrecy, they often had good reason to fear the responses of friends and family members or needed to consider their own vulnerability at this time. The session focused, therefore, on how to decide to disclose to someone important and how to assess both their reactions and one's own readiness. Members helped each other gauge the risks and benefits of coming out to particular individuals and used role plays to act out possible scenarios.

By the ninth session, all the group members had participated in relevant social activities together or with other friends such as going to movies, concerts, bars, dances, art exhibits, etc. During the previous weeks, the women had also spontaneously brought in books, tapes, notices of public events, and resources and had passed these around in the group. In order to build on these experiences, the members first discussed what the notion of community meant to them and came up not only with places and activities with compatible people, but concepts of support, meaning, and personal fulfillment. They then worked in small groups to invent a month in the life of a fictitious lesbian who lived, as far as humanly possible, within the lesbian/gay or women's communities. It was a light-hearted session, but it also revealed to the women that, at least in a large city like Toronto, it is possible to live, work, and find social, spiritual, and recreational activities within the lesbian community a great deal of the time.

GROUP PROCESS ISSUES

All three Women's Coming Out Groups went through the usual stages of group development identified in social group work literature, that is, preaffiliation, power and control, intimacy, differentiation, and separation (Garland, Jones and Kolodny, 1978). Particular issues that were perhaps inevitable in a group of this kind and that added complexity to the group dynamics will be described.

The first incident arose around the third or fourth session and reflected both power and control, and intimacy issues. The group members had shared a great deal of very sensitive and intimate information in telling their "coming out stories" and were simultaneously beginning to socialize on their own. One woman related that, for her, there was a sense of dissonance between what could be talked about in the group and what could be talked about outside. This had come about because she had been teased by another member in a restaurant about something she had said in the group. Initially, this complaint produced great anxiety and panic in the group, with the woman who had made the mistake running out of the room in tears and refusing to return. But the incident also provided a catalyst for members to support both women and to discuss, in a more general way, how to manage the speeded-up kind of intimacy that occurs in a group compared to the slower pace of friendship in more natural settings.

The other issue was that of group members becoming sexually involved. Although there had been a suggestion by the worker that it would be best to postpone such relationships until the conclusion of the group, some women did begin romantic relationships with various consequences for the group and the individuals concerned. In one of the groups where this issue came up, two of the women shyly revealed at the beginning of the sixth session that they had become lovers. The rest of the group responded very warmly, apparently encouraged and inspired by the fact that two of their members had become involved. The following week, another couple declared itself and, all of a sudden, the response changed from one of delight to one of anger and depression.

As the discussion deepened, it became clear that the women who were not in a couple relationship had started to feel threatened by the pairing off that was happening. They feared the breakup of the social group which by now had become very important to them; they worried that the couples would no longer be interested in having other friends; and some felt lonely and inadequate because they did not have a partner. Despite reassurances from the women who were in couples that they had no intention of abandoning their friends, there remained considerable discomfort in the group.

The session on sexuality was more self-conscious and awkward than it might otherwise have been because of the sexual involvement of these two couples. By this time also, one couple had already broken up, and both women said privately that it had been very hard to continue attending group knowing that their former lover was there. On the evaluation sheets, all the women who had been lovers during the group stressed that it would have been better to have waited. This advice was subsequently passed on to the next group by the worker, but to no avail as another pair of women became involved.

Clearly, this is one of the complications of a group in which women who are coming out, and feeling lonely and alienated, suddenly find themselves in a positive environment with other lesbians. Where they are also seeing each other socially and forming authentic and lasting relationships, it is not surprising that some will want to become lovers. This dynamic does, however, present a challenge to the members and the worker as alliances and loyalties can shift and change almost overnight.

Finally, a comment should be made on the general emotional tone in the group. It was very evident that most of the women in all three groups experienced tremendous mood swings from week to week, or even every few days, which they described as "being on an emotional roller coaster." In the worker's experience, this pattern was more pronounced than in other groups, even in coming out groups for adolescents. The group itself was able to normalize this up-and-down process and even to anticipate it in the check-ins. "You were feeling great last week; bet you're a mess this time!" The alternating pattern of vulnerability and strength, despair and hope is perhaps explained by the fact that for most of the women their whole sense of identity was under siege; their beliefs about themselves and relationships with others were undergoing massive redefinition; and, at the same time, life was opening up with new meanings and new possibilities.

Attendance in the Women's Coming Out Groups was extremely high. In the ceremony at the end and in the evaluations, the women consistently talked about the difference that being in the group had made to their whole sense of themselves and feeling of connection with other lesbians. In fact, several said that they had felt "stuck" or "lost" in a general sense for a long time and that now they could go on with their lives. For many women, the group was the crucible in which the painful work of reconstructing an identity and understanding its social context could begin. Coming Out Groups for women continued to be offered two years later, with new leadership and long waiting lists.

REFERENCES

Alissi, S. "The Social Group Work Method: Toward a Reaffirmation of Essentials." Third Annual Symposium on the Advancement of Social Work with Groups. Hartford, Connecticut, October, 1981.

Cass, V. "Homosexuality Identity Formation: A Theoretical Model. " *Journal of Homosexuality,* 1979, *4*(4), 219-221, 1979.

Coleman, E. "Developmental Stages of the Coming Out Process." *American Behavioral Scientist, 24*(4), 426-484, 1982.

Coleman, E. *Integrated Identity for Gay Men and Lesbians: Psychotherapeutic Approaches for Emotional Well-Being.* New York: Harrington Park Press, 1988.

Espin, O. "Issues of Identity in the Psychology of Latina Lesbians." In *Lesbian Psychologies: Explorations and Challenges.* The Boston Lesbian Psychologies Collective (Eds.). Chicago: University of Illinois Press, 1987.

Frye, M. "A Lesbian Perspective on Women's Studies." Presentation given at the National Women's Studies Association Conference. Los Angeles, CA, Spring, 1980.

Fulani, L. (Ed.). Introductory Remarks. *Women and Therapy, 6*(4), 1987.

Garland, J., Jones, H. and Kolodny, R. "Model for Stages in Development in Social Work Groups." In *Explorations in Groupwork: Essays in Theory and Practice.* Hebron, CT: Practitioners Press, 1978.

Gitterman, A. "Building Mutual Support in Groups." *Social Work with Groups, 12*(2), 1989.

Glassman, U. and Kates, L. *Groupwork: A Humanistic Approach.* London: Sage, 1990.

Goffman, E. Stigma: *Notes on the Management of Spoiled Identity.* Harmondsworth: Penguin, 1963.

Jeffreys, S. *Anticlimax: A Feminist Perspective on the Sexual Revolution.* London: The Women's Press, 1990.

Kitzinger, C. *The Social Construction of Lesbianism.* London: Sage Publications, 1987.

Lewis, E. "Regaining Promise: Feminist Perpectives for Social Group Work." Ninth Annual Symposium on Social Work with Groups, Boston, Massachusetts, October, 1987.

Loewenstein, S. "Understanding Lesbian Women." *Social Casework.* January, 29-38, 1980.

Lorde, A. "I am Your Sister: Black Women Organizing Across Sexualities." In *Women and Therapy: The Politics of Race and Gender in Therapy,* L. Fulani, (Ed.), 6(4), 1987.

Middleman, R. and Goldberg, G. "Toward the Quality of Social Group Work Practice." In *Roots and New Frontiers in Social Group Work.* Binghamton: Haworth Press, 1988.

de Monteflores, C. and Schultz, S. "Coming Out: Similarities and Differences for Lesbians and Gay Men." *Journal of Social Issues, 34*(3), 1978.

Pharr, S. *Homophobia: A Weapon of Sexism.* Inverness, CA: Chardon Press, 1988.

Rich, A. "Compulsory Heterosexuality and Lesbian Existence," *Signs: A Journal of Women in Culture and Society.* Summer, 631-57, 1980.

Rothblum, E. and Cole, E. (Eds.). *Loving Boldly: Issues Facing Lesbians.* New York: Harrington Park Press, 1989.

Zitter, S. "Coming Out to Mom." In *Lesbian Psychologies: Explorations and Challenges.* The Boston Lesbian Psychologies Collective (Eds.). Chicago: University of Illinois Press, 1987.

Chapter 9

Being Non-Deliberative on "A Hot Winter's Night": Confessions of a Creative Practitioner

Paul Earl Rivers

The art of social work has to do with mobilizing the creative within the social worker (and the agency) in an effort to foster the creative in the client.

–B. Wheeler
(cited in H. H. Weissman, 1990, p. 275)

SUBSTANTIVE ISSUE

As of March 1991, it had been estimated that 50,000 Canadians were infected with the Human Immunodeficiency Virus (HIV) believed to cause AIDS, and five to ten million people have been infected worldwide. Of these, 650,000 have already developed AIDS, the most severe stage of infection (4768 cases reported in Canada, with 1858 in Ontario alone), and the World Health Organization estimates that the number of AIDS cases will increase nine times in the 1990s (Health and Welfare Canada, 1991).

Education and counseling are essential components in preventing further HIV infection. Without educational campaigns that target persons who engage in unsafe sex for reasons other than lack of accurate information, one can expect to see new cases of HIV infection even among people who have previously been educated about AIDS prevention. Silvestre et al. (1989), for example, report that men who had learned how to avoid HIV infection, and had successfully done so for a time, had knowingly engaged in unsafe behaviors because of either strong emotional responses to certain partners or mental health or drug and alcohol-related problems.

In addition to wide-scale AIDS education campaigns, Kelly and St. Lawrence (1990) discuss the positive impact of community-based skills-training groups (see also Kelly et al., 1989, 1990) and stress that interventions are needed that can directly assist in the development of skills to reduce HIV infection risk behaviors. Skills training and strategies for negotiating condom use in the context of building an intimate relationship need to be explored, and strategies for being assertive with partners who may exert emotional, psychological, or physical pressure to behave unsafely need to be taught. Further, it is unrealistic to assume that all gay and bisexual men will avoid anal intercourse, and instruction in effective decision making about anal intercourse is needed.

Certainly, one sure way to stop the spread of the HIV virus is to engage in safer sex practices. This is difficult to accomplish, however, with just talk or printed material. Cognitive-behavioral and skills-training approaches have helped individuals learn to change other behavior patterns related to health and can be applied to AIDS. Several approaches (i.e., self-management skills training, assertiveness training, and problem solving) are applicable to HIV risk-reduction counseling. Interventions can assist individuals to acquire, use, and maintain behavioral skills that can durably modify risk level. Involvement in multiple-session behavioral group intervention, for example, can produce rapid and clinically meaningful change in high-risk behavior patterns.

SOCIAL WORK PRACTICE EPISODE

Groupwork dilemmas faced in methods of sexuality education with health professionals (Ephross and Weiss, 1985) and adolescents (Cherney and Inclan, 1980) are similar to the one faced on "A Hot Winter's Night": How to eroticize safer sex and teach important facts about AIDS and safer sex to adults without boring them, frightening them, or turning them off. This chapter will describe non-deliberative forms of practice developed and employed by the author in an attempt to address and resolve this groupwork dilemma.

"A Hot Winter's Night" refers to the title for a workshop series on safer sex that was cofacilitated by the author and was intended to change the sex attitudes and practices of participants. Funded by the AIDS Committee of London, it was a teaching/helping endeavor that illustrated an effective, dynamic social work approach to learning and contained several elements of non-deliberative practice.

The goals, purpose, and general principles of "A Hot Winter's Night" were as follows:

1. To eroticize safer sex practices in order to make them preferable to unsafe sexual activity and to identify means by which to realize such practices.
2. To examine the nature of unsafe sexual activity and the emotional and social circumstances that promote it in order to enhance informed choice for safer sex and to identify means of preventing or exiting unsafe sexual situations.
3. To foster a commitment to safer sex practices in order to establish them as long-term behavior change and to identify means of actively promoting safer sex practices for others.

The format consisted of a time-limited (eight sessions) small group (eight to ten participants), as it has been demonstrated that both attitudes and behavior can be effectively changed in the small group format. Each session was two and one-half hours in length and was divided by a short break between a segment that introduced didactic content and a segment that facilitated reflection and response. A multimodal group approach was employed that focused on the following: didactic multi media presentations; experiential exercises, including guided imagery; and the development of a mutual aid system that promoted shared problem-solving, mutual accountability, and personal contracting regarding safer sex practices. Each group had two cofacilitators responsible for presenting the didactic content, fostering the mutual aid system and facilitating self-disclosure and discussion.

MAJOR FEATURES OF THIS FORM OF PRACTICE

It has been clearly demonstrated through the work of sex educators that education that aims at changing attitudes and behavior must be ongoing and interactive (i.e., Kelly et al., 1990). A workshop environment of sufficient duration was needed, then, to cause changes in attitudes, obtain education and allow for experimentation and discussion with knowledgeable facilitators who could successfully eroticize safer sex. It was recognized that such education must deal with emotional issues that affect behavior rather than focus strictly on facts, no matter how explicit. Further, such education must be positive and enticing in presentation rather than negative or guilt or fear inspiring, in order to have the longest impact.

Skills groups, in general, are noted to be behavior-oriented with a focus on the development of specific behaviors and the elimination of self-defeating actions (in this case, life-threatening behavior). Similar to the skills groups discussed by Middleman (1981), this form of practice involved constructed experiences (exercises or simulations) that instructed inductively within the thinking, feeling, and doing domains of learning. The participant was viewed as a "normal" (Middleman, 1981, p. 186) learner, and the worker was the facilitator who acted as the expert in a particular content area and played an active role in pre-planning the format and sequenced sessions as well as in offering brief lectures of theoretical and informational content. Focus was on the here-and-now with a high level of worker control and a high degree of structure.

Additional features of this type of practice included (1) working contractually with participants; (2) specifying goals and procedures for their attainment; (3) using self/other observation as an instructional and evaluative tool; (4) direct practice and drill in various skills and activities; (5) coleadership; and (6) homework assignments intended to link, intensify, or generalize themes to other situations. "Serious play" (Weissman, 1990) was involved through the use of role plays and other constructed experiences in order to provide stimulus for learning adaptive responsiveness with other participants that could be analogous and transferred to "back-home situations" (Middleman, 1981, p. 191).

NON-DELIBERATIVE THEORETICAL
CONNECTIONS

Non-deliberative practice is based on a "do and then think" (Lang, 1992) paradigm in which the worker effects the client's world in some way and experience precedes knowledge. This form of practice has been defined by Lang (1992) as

> A significant experience occurring in a natural form or in a mixed action and participant form, individualized to meet the needs of participants, involving the use of analogues occurring in the context of a significant set of socialization or helping relationships located in and not necessarily abstracted from present reality, using the environment as part of the action in which the client is in the executive role and the worker is in an ancillary but participating/facilitating role, employing problem-solving forms which involve non-rational, non-linear, pre-conscious, creative, analogic, unarticulated thought processes and the use of pre-existing spontaneously arising and deliberately invented and tailor-made media.

The non-deliberative helping approach employed on "A Hot Winter's Night" was constructed on theoretical materials that illuminate understanding of the multiple ways in which people grow, develop, learn and change. These underlying theoretical materials consider such things as the "bicameral mind" (Jaynes, 1976, p. 122) and right-brain function: (1) intuitive, creative, synthesizing, holistic, spatial, analogic, simultaneous (Rico, 1983); (2) divergent and lateral thinking, nonrational problem solving, and serendipitous discovery (Gelfrand, 1988); (3) "effectance" (Perlman, 1965, p. 47); (4) autonomy and competence (Mallucio, 1974); (5) experiential, self-directed learning (Knowles, 1968; Perlman, 1965; Weick and Pope, 1988); (6) the place of action in human growth and development (Mallucio, 1974); (7) the contribution of socialization relationships (McBroom, 1967); and (8) creativity, invention, and holistic problem solving (Gelfrand, 1988; Weissman, 1990).

Methods of intervention included explicit communication and active teaching and modeling. Specific examples of non-deliberative helping forms and means of problem solving employed include the following:

1. The use of games. Session one, for example, included ice-breaker games such as one in which participants wrote down

their two favorite parts of the body on a folded piece of paper, taped it to their chest, and then allowed other participants to lift the top flap in order to discover the preference. Next, the participants broke into pairs to discuss a favorite food and a most recent mistake.

2. The use of role play. Riessman and Goldfarb (1964) note that role playing has been used in work with alcoholics, drug addicts, and suicidal and psychotic patients. They identify it as an action-oriented, "doing versus talking" (Reissman and Goldfarb, 1964, p. 339) mode of problem solving that involves an integration of role theory in sociology and learning theory in psychology. Role plays were designed for "A Hot Winter's Night" to address negotiating safer sex in a public bar "pick-up" scene and anticipating, avoiding, defusing, and exiting unsafe sexual encounters. One scenario, for example, entailed the following instructions for pairs of participants:

> The two of you are ready to, or have begun to have sex. The "INSERTEE" does not want to have safer sex and is resistant to it while the "INSERTER" in insistent on safer sex in the best possible way. Remember that you have five minutes and decide beforehand if the sex you will be talking about is oral sex or anal sex.

3. The use of creative writing. In agreement with Tuzil (1978), the author's opinion is that "by its very nature, writing encourages the active participation of the client in the problem-solving process" (p. 70). As a personal contribution to the content and structure of the series, the author, thus, invited participants to write a "hot fantasy" that eroticized safer sex. Participants were then asked to share the story with other participants at the beginning of a group session following the initial check-in.

As figurative language that is descriptive and emotive in nature has been identified as one variety of verbal language that is analogic (Watzlawick, Weakland, and Fisch, 1974), the "hot fantasy" exercise was a client-created activity that had the potential to become an analog for real-life sexual encounters (e.g., if the client can successfully fantasize about a safer sex encounter, then they can create and experience one in real life). Feedback was positive, and this technique was evaluated as a useful non-deliberative form of practice. The author was pleased to hear that this tradition has continued on subsequent "hot winter's nights," and that the idea of having some of the stories published in a book form is being considered.

Further non-deliberative methods employed include: (1) experiencing safer sex erotica (e.g., videos, written material); (2) relaxation exercises (e.g., guided fantasies); (3) sensual icebreakers (e.g., describing in pairs an experience involving the senses that gives one great pleasure); (4) other experiential exercises of sensate and fantasy nature (e.g., letting a partner move his/her hands in front of one's face while one's eyes are closed, and giving a partner a back-rub in a way one would like to have it done); and (5) homework assignments consisting of personal journals regarding knowledge, feelings, and behavior in relation to workshop material and exercises.

CONCLUSION

A review of literature in theory and research of problem solving reveals that authors have long advocated the use of problem solving as a treatment in behavior modification. Gelfrand (1988), for example, offers a creative problem-solving model that joins the theory and practice of problem solving with the theory and practice of creativity. Creativity is considered necessary when confronted with an unusual or unique situation, and the work of social work requires a creative problem solving approach: human problems are complex, almost impossible to sort out as to causalities, and frequently resistant to change efforts.

Creative, non-deliberative forms of practice can provide one the opportunity for support for taking initiative, respectfully considering ideas, expecting competence and capability as a learner, and having the freedom to experiment and take risks. The author firmly supports the belief that humans have a strong and inevitable impulse toward progression, a belief that underlies this form of practice (Perlman, 1967). Noting that enjoyment sustains creative effort and that the creative person is able to structure experience to maximize pleasure, it is the author's opinion that there exists a definite place for artistry in the use of imaginative and intuitive modes of expression and thought in social work. An internal motivator, the desire for pleasure or enjoyment, recognizes a basic social work issue: give a person a choice and that person will enjoy the activity.

Working inductively "from the experience out" (Lee, 1979, p. 132), the author notes that deliberate attempts were made on "A Hot Winter's Night" to seduce learners to venture new behaviors and, therefore, expand their repertoire of sensual and safer sexual responses. This skills group effectively used non-deliberative forms of practice to promote competence through a learning opportunity that focused on action, information getting, achievement of comfort vis-à-vis others and the environment, and the experience of options and choices. Noting that the process of learning occurs most readily when learners are "relaxed and involved . . . open and risking" (Maier, 1980, p. 7), a group milieu was created to reflect a climate for learning (i.e., physical set-up of chairs in a circle, safer sex-related posters displayed on the walls).

Whereas Weissman (1990) stated that "creativity begins with doubt and questions . . . when practitioners doubt the value of their work or question the methods they are using" (p. 27), the author, as a participant in the initial pilot series, did have some concerns about the high level of structure and worker control. It was these concerns, in fact, that inspired the innovative idea to add a self-directed "Hot Fantasy" exercise to the structure and content of the skills group. With pride, the author recalls to this date several images and fantasies that would heat up the coldest of winter nights.

REFERENCES

Cherney, M. J. and Inclan, R. (1980). An Effective Method of Teaching Facts Within a Groupwork Context. *Social Work with Groups, 3* (1), 17-21.

Ephross, P. and Weiss, J. (1985). The Use of Group Methods in Sexuality Education for Health Professions. *Social Work with Groups, 8*(3), 59-69.

Gelfrand, B. (1988). *The Creative Practitioner: Creative Theory and Method for the Helping Services.* Binghamton: The Haworth Press.

Health and Welfare Canada. (1991). *Aids in the 90's: The New Facts of Life.* (Publication No. ISBN 0-919245-42-0). Ottawa: Queen's Printer for Ontario.

Jaynes, J. (1976). *The Origin of Consciousness in the Breakdown of the Bicameral Mind.* Boston: Houghton Mifflin.

Kelly, J. A. and St. Lawrence, J. S. (1990). The Impact of Community-Based Groups to Help Persons Reduce HIV Infection Risk behaviors. *AIDS Care, 2* (1), 25-36.

Kelly, J. A., St. Lawrence, J. S., Betts, R., Brasfield, T. L., et. al. (1990). A Skills-Training Group Intervention Model to Assist Persons in Reducing Risk behaviors for HIV Infection. *AIDS Education and Prevention, 2*(1), 24-35.

Kelly, J. A., St. Lawrence, J. S., Hood, H. V., and Brasfield, T. L. (1989). Behavioral Intervention to Reduce AIDS Risk Activities. *Journal of Consulting and Clinical Psychology, 57*(1), 60-67.

Knowles, M. (1968). Andragogy, Not Pedagogy. *Adult Leadership, 16*(10), 350-352, 368.

Lang, N. C. (1992). Course material. Non-Deliberative Forms of Practice in Social Work. Toronto: University of Toronto.

Lee, J. A. (1979). The Foster Parents Workshop: A Social Work Approach to Learning for New Foster Parents. *Social work with Groups, 2*(2), 129-143.

Maier, H. W. (1980). Play in the University Classroom. *Social Work with Groups, 3*(1), 7-16.

Mallucio, T. (1974). Action as a Tool in Casework Practice. *Social Casework, LV,* 30-35.

McBroom, E. (1967). The Socialization of Parents. *Child Welfare, LVI,* 132-136.

Middleman, R. R. (1981). The Pursuit of Competence Through Involvement in Structured Groups. In A. N. Maluccio (Ed.). *Promoting Competence in Clients* (pp. 185-210). New York: Free Press.

Perlman, H. H. (1967). . . . And Gladly Teach. *Journal of Education for Social Work, 3*(1), 41-50.

Perlman, H. H. (1965). Self-Determination: Reality or Illusion? *Social Service Review,* December, 125-145.

Rico, G. L. (1983). *Writing the Natural Way: Using Right-Brain Techniques to Release Your Expressive Powers.* Boston: Houghton Mifflin Company.

Riessman, F. and Goldfarb, J. (1964). Role Playing and the Poor. In F. Riessman, J. Cohen, and A. Pearl (Eds.). *Mental Health of the Poor* (pp. 336-347). New York: Free Press.

Silvestre, A. J., Lyter, D. W., Vadiserri, R. O., Huggins, J., and Rinaldo Jr., R. (1989). Factors Related to Seroconversion Among Homo- and Bisexual Men After a Risk- Reduction Educational Session. *AIDS,* 3(10), 647-650.

Tuzil, T. J. (1978). Writing: A Problem-Solving Process. *Social Work, 23*(1), 67-70.

Watzlawick, P., Weakland, S., and Fisch, R. (1974). *Change: Principles of Problem Formulation and Resolution.* New York: Norton.

Weick, A. and Pope, L. (1988). Knowing What's Best: A New Look at Self-Determination. *Social Casework, 69*(1), 10-16.

Weissman, H. H. (1990). *Serious Play: Creativity & Innovation in Social Work.* Silver Spring, MD: NASW.

Chapter 10

Trauma Debriefings:
A One-Session Group Model

Tom Reynolds
Gwyn Jones

During the last five years in the employee assistance program (EAP) field, in Canada, there has been a dramatic increase in the use of debriefing as a way of dealing with traumatic events that occur at the workplace. Canadian EAP companies have been able to heighten the awareness of organizations regarding victims of a traumatic event. Proponents of debriefing models believe that individuals who do not have the opportunity to express their feelings about the impact of an event do carry excess emotional baggage (Davis and Friedman, 1985).

As clinicians, we are aware that frightening circumstances or events can occur, without warning, in any of our lives. When those circumstances are seen as potentially life-threatening to ourselves or others, or if they challenge the stability of our relationships, our work, home environments, or our communities, these circumstances could easily be viewed as a *critical incident*, or a *traumatic occurrence*.

Much of the literature written in the area of trauma or critical incidents concurs with the belief that an early therapeutic intervention is "very effective in reducing critical incident stress or long-term effects of trauma" (Manton and Talbot, 1990). Warren Shepell Consultants has been providing therapeutic interventions, known as *Trauma Response Services,* on an ad hoc basis to organizational clients through its employee assistance program since 1985. In 1989, our involvement in the field grew with our contract to provide

129

trauma response services to employees of a major national bank in response to helping individuals who were involved in bank holdups.

The purpose of the service as stated in our policy and procedures manual is as follows:

1. To normalize employee/s reactions to the traumatic event and educate them in the area of post trauma reactions.
2. To support the employee/s and facilitate a discussion of their emotional reaction(s) to the traumatic event.
3. To provide active listening that enhances understanding of and gives meanings to the employee/s experiences.
4. To reduce the potential long-term impact of the event on the employee's professional and personal life.

The design of debriefing sessions seems to have been influenced by models described in the literature during the last decade. The literature describes the practice of professionals who offered services to victims after events like major community disasters (i.e., the University of Montreal massacre, Montreal, 1989; the MGM Hotel fire, Las Vegas, 1980; the Hyatt Skywalk collapse, Kansas City, 1981). In 1980, the American Psychiatric Association formally recognized a new syndrome, calling it the posttraumatic stress disorder (PTSD). Debriefings have tended to focus either on individual stress reactions or on the prevention of the disorder in individuals. Recognition of the power of the group has been acknowledged by way of using groups to debrief, with the emphasis on a psychoeducational approach.

Based on some of the literature and also on our own experiences, some group leaders would claim to be responsive to group needs by enabling individuals to vent and share feelings with each other. However, it is our contention that in order to maximize the full potential and resources of a one session group, the worker must be knowledgeable in groupwork theory (phases, contracting, leadership, etc.) as well as competent in groupwork practice.

In this chapter, we will explore the use of a debriefing as a one-session group model. We will share our experiences of these groups as having similar properties to those groups that are longer term, and examine how leaders make use of these properties in order to maximize the work done by a group in a limited time frame. In other words, the group worker in a single session faces the challenge of guiding the group through various phases, while respecting the integrity of the group processes. Worker ability to establish contact and maintain it as a thread in the group's development is a key factor in the accomplishment of the group's task.

STAGES OF A TRAUMA DEBRIEFING MODEL

There have been a variety of frameworks used to describe phases in groupwork development (Garland, Jones, and Kolodny, 1973; Northen, 1969; Shulman, 1984). For the purpose of this chapter, we will discuss the trauma debriefing group phases as the following: (1) pre-group; (2) beginning; (3) middle; (4) ending; and (5) post-group phases.

Pre-Group Activity

The goal of this phase is to organize the beginning session. This is accomplished by discussion with the manager of the workgroup or an individual with authority to bring the group together. The issues to be attended to are those common to pre-group activity in most groups. For example, composition and size, length, time and location, intake data, such as nature of event, intensity of the event, and observed impact on the organization are all things to be considered.

Assessments of potential group members are done by telephone. They are conducted primarily with the manager, with input as needed from other staff members. The purpose is to screen out anyone not appropriate for group intervention. The prospective group members are familiar with this form of pre-group assessment and with the likelihood of their being included in the debriefing group. There is an important balancing act to be done in gathering information and facts about the event without co-opting the manager into a coleadership role that may not be useful in the actual debriefing session. For instance, the manager may give impressions of employees' mental states, and try to give advice about whom to focus on in the group. It is important to listen and respond in a way that joins, and does not serve to distance, from the other employees or the manager to the group as a whole.

A major skill in the preliminary phase of work is the development of the worker's preparatory empathy. Schwartz terms this as tuning in and involves the worker's efforts to get in touch with the potential feelings and concerns that any client may bring to the helping encounter (Schwartz and Zalba, 1971). The manager may show signs of guilt and feelings of responsibility for the occurrence which may be out of proportion to the actual event. The worker or leader in this phase must be able to listen, normalize, and validate the manager's experience as well as to enhance awareness of the shared nature of that experience (i.e., other employees may be feeling similar things). The task of the pre-group phase is to educate the manager about what will take place at the debriefing session. Because the manager's collaboration is crucial at this point, it is extremely important that this intervention be seen as a meaningful and productive process. The decision, whether or not to go ahead with the session, is at the manager's discretion. It is timely to emphasize the importance of group leaders joining with the hierarchy of the organizations whom they serve. However, the risk at this stage is de-emphasizing a manager's group membership role by over-utilizing that manager as a source of specialized knowledge of the organization and of the event.

Beginning Phase

During this phase a number of tasks are carried out. The primary and most important is the contracting task. The ability of the worker to negotiate the purpose and goals of the group will determine the extent to which it is successful. The leader of the trauma debriefing session explains very clearly what his idea is about the format of the group, the length of time available, and what he thinks will be the work of the group. This then is negotiated with the members of the group by facilitating discussion about what expectations they have about the session. Often members' ideas vary from thinking that the session may be used as a management tool in order to reprimand employees for their handling of the trauma, to fearing that the group leader is there in order to ascertain which of the employees are most in need of help from the EAP service.

In this stage, the main dynamics are the safety of each individual, the approach and avoidance dilemma for each individual and a general exploration of the group itself as mentioned previously (Nosko and Wallace, 1988). The worker/leader must take care in assuring the group about confidentiality. This is often a dilemma as the manager is also a group participant, however, what happens in the group is not shared with any individuals in the organization outside this group. There is often a distrust with some members about the limitations of this confidentiality with the manager present. This necessitates the worker's sensitively encouraging the manager to respond to these verbal or nonverbal requests. The clarification and negotiation of these issues are often the basis of the group's working together and accomplishing the group tasks.

For example, in organizing the group debriefing, the EAP worker/leader coaches the manager regarding confidentiality issues. A typical manager's statement regarding confidentiality would be "I've invited EAP here today to help us with what happened. As you know, EAP has strict confidentiality, that is, what you say here will go no further than this room. EAP will not tell (other) management, or anyone else for that matter, what is said. It is important that you know that so that you can feel safe to talk if you want to." Managers often leave at this point, unless they were actually involved in the incident. This process is important because it delivers two very significant messages:

1. By being present and introducing the meeting, the manager makes a statement indicating support and endorsement of the process, and
2. Whether by leaving or staying the manager is modeling respect for confidentiality.

Because of the time limitation of the session, the worker frequently is more directive than he would be in a multi-session group. The leader states what he or she is there to do and what he or she is not going to do. For example, leaders may reach for some of the preconceptions that the employees may have, and explain that they will ask about their experiences of the event and the subsequent time period. They share that they will provide information about the kinds of reactions people normally have and explain that there will be a discussion of the kinds of activity that help relieve the symptom. They reassure the members that participation is voluntary and that they will not single out people should they choose not to enter into discussions. The worker also informs the group that there will be an opportunity to meet individually with the leader/worker following the group session.

It is important to note here that one goal for these post group meetings is to allow for an assessment of high-risk individuals. EAP professionals who are trained to look for the signs of post traumatic stress disorder can then see to it that its sufferers are quickly referred to treatment. This can help resolve a potentially chronic problem, restore valuable human resources, and save thousands of dollars that would otherwise be lost to payments for disability, treatment, rehabilitation, and litigation.

The tasks described above are done through a process of discussion, negotiation, and compromise. As an example, some groups have the flexibility to negotiate a longer time with the leader. The leader works with the members and manager, and, if the organizational context permits, the time frame may be extended to one and one-half to two hours. Some managers wish to exclude themselves from the group session in order to give employees greater freedom to express themselves. All of these kinds of issues are worked out in this stage.

Clarity of the contractual agreements is a critical role of the worker/leader. If there is lack of structure and/or absence of clearly defined and accepted rules of behavior, then the stage is set for the group to sabotage the work. With the contract agreed upon, the group is now ready to face the tasks associated with the power and control, intimacy, and differential stages of the group (Garland, Jones, and Kolodny, 1973).

The Middle Phase

The worker, because of the time restrictions, is active in helping the group move from a beginning phase to the middle phase (Rotholz, 1985). Usually at this phase the members feel safer with each other and, to some degree, with the leader. In many ways, the members of the groups with which we work know each other outside of the group session. This can help move the group more quickly (Block, 1985). We certainly do notice this to be operating in this stage as members start to challenge other members. Very early in some groups, we have found that members may disagree with another as they describe the sequence of traumatic events. "That's not what happened Bill, you had your eyes closed most of the time the robber was there"; or, "I disagree with you Mary, I think you are upset. You haven't been able to focus on your job since it happened." Members will also test the worker. "What good is talking about this anyway? It won't help." Questions of competency and adequacy are likely to be upsetting for the worker if he is not expecting it. Members may also trigger issues of authority for the worker and how his authority can be used. This may create some anxiety if the worker has unresolved issues around authority or fears of losing control of the group. At times like these we have seen some leaders revert to a more didactic format and use less process. They tend to steer around the issues and see the challenging as disruptive, rather than view it as a normal and healthy aspect of group development.

The group leader asks employees/members of the group to recall the event. In order to elicit this information, questions are directed to the group as a whole rather than to a particular individual. Through a series of questions designed to avoid the stigma of self-disclosure, members are invited to talk about the reactions, thoughts, feelings, and physiological responses. As the group approaches intense emotional material, a common group dynamic seen is scapegoating. In one group, a member who was perceived by many members as less intelligent and competent shared that her reaction to the trauma after she went home was to look under the bed and in the closets. The group responded by lots of laughter and whispering that isolated the member from the other alliances in the group. The worker helped the group explore their use of scapegoating as a way of avoiding their own emotions about the trauma.

The leader guides employees along a time continuum from the start of the traumatic event to the experience of coming to work the very morning of the group session. Members are also helped to recall previous traumas in their lives, as well as to explore their fantasies regarding a perilous future. Various groupwork interventions are used: (1) modeling; (2) self-disclosure; (3) norm-setting; (4) conflict exploration; (5) exploration of metacommunication patterns including investigating silence; and (6) information giving. In this way, a more autonomous system is set up, enabling therapeutic group and subgroup interactions to continue beyond the end of this single session and into their regular working context. The establishment of a mutual aid system like this has largely been discussed in the literature in the context of a longer term multisession model rather than a singlesession model (Glassman and Kates, 1990).

The Ending Phase

The transition to this phase illustrates the need for the group leader to shift roles and activities quickly and with flexibility (Block, 1985). The leader helps the members identify resources outside the group to which they can be connected. Since this is already a group with previous connections, it is likely some members will be strengthened by the group experience and become more able to access each other for support outside the group. Waldron, in her article describing one-session groups with children whose parents are in the military, emphasizes that the previous connections of the children outside the group strengthen the impact of the limited group experience (Waldron, Whittington, and Jensen, 1985).

The leader reviews some relevant points that were shared through the process of the group, such as the natural reactions they may yet encounter and experience, and strategies for alleviating symptoms. The members are also given a handout by the leader to take with them. During the ending phase, the worker/leader reinforces the options available to group members to meet with the worker individually after the group session closes.

The move to a more pragmatic approach serves to decrease the intensity of the group as the leader becomes more active and central. Termination stage includes the worker's reaching for members' feelings and experiences about the group. Members at times raise their disappointment that not all their questions were answered, and not all solutions to deal with their reactions and fears were discussed. This is consistent to ending phases of groups when members deny the ending and try to re-engage the worker into prolonging the group (i.e., going overtime). The worker leads strives to help them connect to a life beyond the group–their supports with each other, their families and friends, the EAP services, etc.

Post-Group Phase

This phase normally has two activities. First, the leader will give group members the opportunity to meet with him or her individually following the group session. One goal has already been mentioned and that is for trained EAP professionals to look for signs of PTSD and make a referral. This procedure is one that is guided by each worker's assessment of the uniqueness of each context. It is seen as important for each employee to have a few minutes with the worker in order to allow opportunities for the employee to raise questions, share information and feelings that the member may not have felt comfortable expressing within the group. The worker might be especially attentive to this if the event involved a high degree of violence. Workers are especially sensitive to the employee's readiness and willingness to use this session and also respectful of an employee's wish to keep the meeting brief. The group worker gives a card with the EAP telephone number on it, should the employee want to access service following the meeting.

Second, the worker or trauma service coordinator reactivates contact with the manager by phone several days later. The goals are to elicit feedback from the manager about how his staff experienced the group and to offer the availability of ongoing counseling, if required. The worker, or trauma service coordinator must avoid co-opting the manager into a postgroup leadership role.

CONCLUSION

The single session approach to delivering trauma services to organizations is utilized for a variety of reasons. Primarily, in the case of doing a group in a bank after a 'holdup,' the nature of the organization dictates an immediate, brief approach. The debriefing sessions are usually held before working hours so that all staff involved in the traumatic event can attend. There is sensitivity to the fact that the bank must also open its doors even after such a difficult occurrence. Providing the debriefing session so quickly to all staff indicates a responsiveness on the part of the organization's management to the needs of the employees. We have done surveys on the value of the debriefings with the banks. The statistics have indicated the usefulness of this intervention.

Organizations, other than banks, also use this service. As previously mentioned, industrial accidents, major downsizing, assault, accidental deaths, and suicides are situations where the trauma service becomes involved. In these events, a typical debriefing is a one-session group with a longer time frame. This lengthening of the time frame has been found to be useful by clinicians who work with the groups. They feel more can be accomplished, and it also provides a greater ease in working the group through the various phases.

Shulman talks about the reluctance of some workers to use a one-session group model. The reasons range from the groups being too large to the groups having not enough time to do their work. He states that some workers feel that there is too much to cover and therefore not enough time for the group process. Shulman feels firmly that there is great value in the single-session group and that the stage framework is essential to understanding how to make the most of the limited time to do the work of the group (Shulman, 1984).

Our belief is that in providing the trauma debriefings the members are educated about symptoms of critical incident stress, which is helpful in the prevention of serious emotional after-effects. This position is supported by many of the authors describing their single-session models in the literature. However, in our view, the group in the debriefing sessions enters into the most useful terrain as it establishes a mutual aid system. Therefore, it is essential that the leader has this as a goal. It is through this mutual aid system that individual members grow. Through the processes of sharing, being supported, learning from others, being challenged, and having reactions normalized, members usually leave the group with an enhanced perception of themselves. They emerge as coping individuals, a capacity that they may have previously doubted. They also carry forward the values of support and acceptance as opposed to wanting to judge or isolate people experiencing stress.

The use of trauma debriefing after critical incidents is on the increase. It is no longer sufficient to teach practitioners the rudiments of post traumatic stress disorder. For trauma debriefings to be most effective, training must now focus on groupwork theory and practice. Without understanding the power and uniqueness of a group, the authors note that the benefits of the intervention may not endure.

REFERENCES

Block, L. R. "On the Potentiality and the Limits of Time: The Single Session Group and the Cancer Patient." *Social Work with Groups* (Summer): 81-97, 1985.

Davis, R. C. and Freidman, L. N. "The Emotional Aftermath of Crime and Violence." Figley, C.R. (Ed.). *Trauma and Its Wake: The Study and Treatment of Post-Traumatic Stress Disorder.* New York: Brunner Mazel, 1985:90-112.

Garland, J. A., Jones, H. E., and Kolodny, R. L. "A Model for Stages of Development in Social Work Groups." Bernstein, S. (Ed.). *Explorations in Group Work.* Boston: Milford House, 1973:17-71.

Glassman, U. and Kates, L. *Group Work: A Humanistic Approach.* California: Sage, 1990.

Manton, M. and Talbot, A. "Crisis Intervention After an Armed Hold-up: Guidelines for Counsellors." *Journal of Traumatic Stress* (3):507-521, 1990.

Northen, H. *Social Work with Groups.* New York: Columbia University Press, 1969.

Nosko, A. and Wallace, B. "Group Work with Abusive Men: A Multidimensional Model." *Social Work with Groups* (11):33-49, 1985.

Rotholz, T. "The Single Session Group: An Innovative Approach to the Waiting Room." *Social Work with Groups* (Summer):143-145, 1985.

Schwartz, W. "On the Use of Groups in Social Work Practice." Schwartz, W. and Zalba S. (Ed.). *The Practice of Group Work.* New York: Columbia University Press, 1971:3-24.

Shulman, L. *The Skills of Helping Individuals and Groups.* Boston: Peacock, 1984.

Waldron, J. A., Whittington, R. R., and Jensen, S. "Children's Single-Session Debriefings: Group Work with Military Families Experiencing Parents' Development." *Social Work with Groups* (Summer):101-108, 1985.

Index

Page numbers followed by the letter "t" designate tables.

AA (Alcoholics Anonymous), 88-89
Acquired Immunodeficiency
        Syndrome (AIDS)
    epidemiology of, 119
    ethical issues in, 37-38
    future issues in, 42-43
    group work and, 33-43. *See also*
        Persons with AIDS (PWAs),
        groups for
    and identity, 37-39,42
    prevention programs for, 119-126
        behavioral techniques in,
            121-122
        creative writing in, 124-125
        format of, 121
        non-deliberative techniques
            in, 122-125
        role plays in, 124
    and social isolation, 40
Adolescents, African-American,
        group work with, 45-55. *See
        also* African-American
        adolescents
African-American adolescents,
        group work with, 45-55
    dance in, 48-49
    decision making in, 49-53
    interpersonal relationships among,
        51-53
    self-concept in, 47-48
    termination in, 53-54
Afrocentric perspective, 45-46

AIDS. *See* Acquired
        Immunodeficiency
        Syndrome
Alcoholics Anonymous. *See* AA
Alcoholism, in women
    depression and, 90-91
    group work with, 87-99. *See also*
        Recovering women, group
        work with
    victimization and, 90

Behavioral techniques, in AIDS
        prevention programs, 121-122

Cardiac patients, group work
        with spouses of, 64-67
Casework, vs. group work, 25
Clients, group as, 15
Coming out groups, for lesbians,
        103-117. *See also* Lesbians
Community services, for elderly
        persons, 59,59t
Confidentiality
    in coming out groups for lesbians,
        112
    in trauma debriefings, 133
Contracting, in trauma debriefings,
        132
Creative writing, in AIDS prevention
        programs, 124-125
Crisis intervention, in group work
        with recovering women, 94

141

Dance, group work involving, with
     African-American
     adolescents, 48-49
Death, discussion of, in groups for
     persons with AIDS, 40-42
Debriefing, after trauma, 129-139.
     See also Trauma debriefings
Decision-making
   in group work with
        African-American
        adolescents, 49-53
   in student groups, 78. *See also*
        Students
Depression, and alcoholism,
     in women, 90-91
Diabetics, group work with, 62-64

EAPs (employee assistance
     programs), trauma
     debriefings in, 129-139. *See
     also* Trauma debriefings
Ecological model, in group work
     with recovering women,
     91-93
Educational programs, for safer sex,
     119-126. *See also* Acquired
     Immunodeficiency Syndrome
     (AIDS), prevention programs
     for
Elderly persons
   care of, social factors in, 60
   community services for, 59,59t
   demographic changes in, 58-59
Emotional tone, in coming out
     groups for lesbians, 115
Empathy, preparatory, in trauma
     debriefings, 132
Employee assistance programs. *See*
     EAPs
Empowerment model, in group work
     with recovering women,
     93-94
Ethical issues, in Acquired
     Immunodeficiency
     Syndrome, 37-38

Feelings, identification of, in group
     work with recovering
     women, 96-97
Feminist perspective, in coming out
     groups for lesbians, 108-109

Graduate schools, group work
     courses in, 23-24,26,71-84.
     See also Students, group
     work with
Group development, in student
     groups, 81-83
Group members, interpersonal
     relationships among. *See*
     Relationships, among group
     members
Group process issues, in coming out
     groups for lesbians, 114-117
Group work
   Acquired Immunodeficiency
        Syndrome and, 33-43. *See
        also* Acquired
        Immunodeficiency Syndrome
   with adolescents,
        African-American, 45-55.
        See also African-American
        adolescents
   vs. casework, 25
   courses in, 23-24,26,72-84. *See
        also* Students, group work
        with
   in hospitals, 57-69. *See also*
        Hospitals, group work in
   mutual aid in, 25,138
   with oncology staff, 67-68
   perceptions of
        by colleagues, 21-22
        history of, 21
   promotion of, 19-31
        avenues for, 28-31
   with recovering women, 87-99.
        See also Recovering women,
        group work with

Group work *(continued)*
  with students, 71-84. *See also*
    Students, group work with
Groups, "two clients" in, 15

Health care, group work in, 57-69.
    See also Hospitals, group
    work in
Heart disease, group work with
    spouses of patients, 64-67
High-risk assessment, in trauma
    debriefings, 134
Homophobia, 104,113
Hospitals, group work in, 57-69
  with cardiac spouses, 64-67
  with diabetics, 62-64
  for oncology staff, 67-68
Human Immunodeficiency Virus
    (HIV) infection, prevention
    programs for, 119-126. *See
    also* Acquired
    Immunodeficiency Syndrome

Identity
  Acquired Immunodeficiency
    Syndrome and, 37-39,42
  issues concerning, in coming out
    groups for lesbians, 105-107
Interactional paradigm, 7-16
  elements of, 7
  oppression model and, clinical
    example of, 8-15
Interactions, patterns of, in student
    groups, 79-81
Interpersonal relationships, among
    groups members. *See*
    Relationships, among group
    members
Isolation, social
  Acquired Immunodeficiency
    Syndrome and, 40
  in lesbians, 106

Lesbians
  coming out groups for, 103-117
    advantages of, 107-110
    composition of, 110-111
    confidentiality in, 112
    emotional tone of, 115
    feminist perspective in, 108-109
    goals of, 108
    group process issues in, 114-117
    identity issues in, 105-107
    sexual activity among members
      of, 115-116
    structure of, 111-114
    themes in, 111-114
  identity issues in, 105-107
  social isolation in, 106
Life cycle, reenactment of, in groups
    for persons with AIDS, 41-42

Medical model
  in group work with recovering
    women, 88-91
  vs. medical paradigm, 5
Medical paradigm, 2-5
Modern dance, group work
    involving, with African-
    American adolescents, 48-49
Morality model, in group work with
    recovering women, 87-88
Mutual aid, in group work, 25,138

Non-deliberative techniques,
    in AIDS prevention
    programs, 122-125
Norms, in student groups, 76-78

Oncology staff, group work
    with, 67-68
Oppression model, 5-7
  and interactional paradigm,
    clinical example of, 8-15

Paradigms
  definition of, 1-2
  interactional, 7-16. *See also*
    Interactional paradigm
  medical, 2-5
  shifts in, 15-16
Parenting, in group work with
    recovering women, 98
Persons with AIDS (PWAs), groups
    for, 33-43
  discussion of death in, 40-42
  future issues in, 42-43
  life cycle reenactment in, 41-42
Power, in coming out groups
    for lesbians, 115
Pregroup phase, of trauma
    debriefings, 131-132
Preparatory empathy, in trauma
    debriefings, 132
Problem solving, in group work
    with recovering women,
    95-96
PWAs. *See* Persons with AIDS

Recovering women, group work
    with, 87-99
  crisis intervention in, 94
  ecological model in, 91-93
  empowerment model in, 93-94
  evaluation of, 98-99
  feeling identification in, 96
  medical model in, 88-91
  morality model in, 87-88
  parenting in, 98
  problem solving in, 95-96
  relationships in, 97-98
  value of, 94-95
Relationships, among group
    members
  African-American adolescent,
    51-53
  of cardiac spouses, 66
  in recovering women, 97-98

Role plays, in AIDS prevention
    programs, 124
Roles, in student groups, 73-76

Safer sex, educational programs for,
    119-126. *See also* Acquired
    Immunodeficiency Syndrome
    (AIDS), prevention programs
    for
Scapegoating, in trauma debriefings,
    135
Self-concept, skin color and, 47-48
Sexual activity
  among members of coming out
    groups for lesbians, 115-116
  safer, educational programs for,
    119-126. *See also* Acquired
    Immunodeficiency Syndrome
    (AIDS), prevention
    programs, for
Sexual orientation, socialization
    about, 103-104
Skin color, and self-concept, 47-48
Social isolation
  Acquired Immunodeficiency
    Syndrome and, 40
  in lesbians, 106
Socialization
  about sexual orientation, 103-104
  as theme in coming out groups
    for lesbians, 113-114
Spouses, of cardiac patients
  group work with, 64-67
Students,
  decision making in, 78
  evaluation of, 83-84
  group development in, 81-83
  group work with, 71-84
  interactional patterns in, 81-83
  norms in, 76-78
  roles in, 73-76
  subgroups in, 80-81

Termination
  in group for African-American
    adolescents, 53-54
  in trauma debriefings, 136-137
Themes, in coming out groups
    for lesbians, 111-114
Trauma debriefings, 129-139
  beginning phase of, 132-134
  confidentiality in, 133
  contracting in, 132
  effectiveness of, 130
  high-risk assessment in, 134
  middle stage of, 134-136
  post-group stage of, 137
  pregroup phase of, 131-132
  preparatory empathy in, 132

Trauma debriefings *(continued)*
  scapegoating in, 135
  termination phase of, 136-137

Victimization, and alcoholism,
    in women, 90

Women, recovering, group work
    with, 87-99. *See also*
    Recovering women, group
    work with
Writing, creative, in AIDS
    prevention programs, 124